praise for every woman's yoga

"This practical guide, based on the time-honored wisdom of yoga philosophy, will inspire women to move toward wholeness, vitality, and balance in a gentle manner."

—Pandit Rajmani Tigunait, Ph.D., spiritual head,
Himalayan Institute

"Grounded in the most authentic teachings of yoga and happily avoiding the whistles and bells of "brand name yogas," this simple and elegant book will be a joy for the woman who picks it up and works with it regularly."

—Rudolph Ballentine, M.D.,
author of *Radical Healing*

"With firm moorings in traditional yoga, *Every Woman's Yoga* encompasses many of the lofty principles of classical yoga while being extremely practical and useful to every woman."

—Srivatsa Ramaswami, author of
Yoga for the Three Stages of Life

"From strengthening to relaxation to soul connection, Jaime has created a beautifully thorough book for all women at any stage of life."

—Colette Crawford, R.N.,
director of Seattle Holistic Center

"*Every Woman's Yoga* is an excellent guidebook for women of all ages and cultures. Jaime Stover Schmitt has written a masterful work on the ancient, life-generating practice of yoga evoking the feminine spirit of healing and nurturance."

—Swamini Mayatitananda (formerly Bri. Maya
Tiwari), author of *The Path of Practice*

"*Every Woman's Yoga* offers a cornucopia of tried-and-true traditional practices that work and are truly transformational. Jaime Stover Schmitt invites us into a world of yoga that ignites spontaneity."

—Kevin Kortan, yoga therapist and teacher,
and creator of Evolutionary Yoga

"Jamie Stover Schmitt in her book, *Every Woman's Yoga*, offers in a comprehensive and clearly organized way, her understanding of yoga as applied to the special issues of women. This book will be welcomed by women who seek to know themselves more fully and improve their health from within."

—Bonnie Bainbridge Cohen,
founder and educational director,
the School for Body-Mind Centering

every woman's yoga

how to incorporate strength, flexibility, and balance into your life

Jaime Stover Schmitt

PRIMA PUBLISHING

I offer this work at the Feet of the Divine Mother whose Love has guided me through my own beautiful mother, Laura Jane Stover, and through H. H. Sri Mata Amritanandamayi Devi. I offer this work at the Feet of H. H. Sri Swami Rama and the Teachers of the Tradition of the Himalayan Masters.

Published by Prima Publishing, Roseville, California. Member of the Crown Publishing Group, a division of Random House, Inc., New York.

PRIMA PUBLISHING and colophon are trademarks of Random House, Inc., registered with the United States Patent and Trademark Office.

Interior design by Mary Beth Salmon
Illustrations by Roger Hill

"The Guest House" by Rumi from *The Essential Rumi* (translated by Coleman Barks, with John Moyne, A. J. Arberry, and Reynold Nicholson). Reprinted by permission.

Library of Congress Cataloging-in-Publication Data
Schmitt, Jaime Stover.
    Every woman's yoga : how to incorporate strength, flexibility, and balance into
your life / Jaime Stover Schmitt.
        p.   cm.
    Includes index.
    ISBN 0-7615-3722-8
    1. Yoga, Hatha. 2. Women—Health and hygiene. 3. Exercise for women. 4. Yoga.
I. Title.
RA781.7 .S297   2002
613.7'046—dc21   2002074977

02 03 04 05 06 BB 10 9 8 7 6 5 4 3 2 1
Printed in the United States of America

First Edition

Visit us online at www.primapublishing.com

contents

foreword

Modern life encourages us to look outward to find meaning. We are distracted by media, news, and fashion, and many times we don't take the time to find meaning within. Business, the beauty industry, and consumerism dominate society, and therefore tend to rule our minds and lives. We think we will be happy when we measure up to society's standards: Look beautiful and attain significant wealth. But the truth is that we aren't completely happy—even when we do succeed in meeting these goals. That's because we find true joy and peace and purpose when we look inside ourselves. *Every Woman's Yoga*, by Jaime Stover Schmitt, is a user-friendly, comprehensive invitation to do just that. In these frenetic times, this book offers us a welcome respite of clarity, peace, and yogic wisdom.

The practice of yoga is a wonderful way to begin the inward journey. We can start with physical movements and breathing techniques that make us feel more flexible, calm, and healthy. We can also practice meditation and contemplation to help us deal with stress, anxiety, and depression. In a systematic way, yoga offers all the tools we need to explore and understand our entire nature—body, energy, emotions, mind, and spirit. According to the science of yoga, health and happiness come to us when we understand and integrate these parts of ourselves. As Jaime says, "Each yoga practice, whether it emphasizes moving, holding a pose, tending the breath, or focusing the mind, invites you to integrate body, breath, mind, and emotions." This is the foundation of health and well-being.

For this reason, *Every Woman's Yoga* is essential (as the title says!) to *every* woman—young or old, a beginner at yoga or a more practiced student. As a beginning yoga manual, it teaches standard yoga poses, breathing, and relaxation to help you stretch, get in shape, and destress. It is also a guide for those seeking to deepen or refresh their current practice by listening to the voice of the body. Jaime includes numerous variations and practical tips about poses, as well as ways to make your yoga practice work for you. Her message is consistently, "Listen within." Your practice, she says, should be molded to suit you, rather than you molding yourself to suit your yoga practice. Your practice shouldn't be another "should" that you aren't quite doing right! Rather you should feel better in body and mind every time you practice—not exhausted, but refreshed and revitalized.

On a personal level, Jaime has been an inspiration in my life. As a colleague, teacher, and friend, I have witnessed over and over her devotion to helping others heal through this integrative work. She speaks with the knowledge gleaned from over two decades of experience in teaching yoga in groups and to individual clients and from developing her own practice. What I admire most about Jaime is her absolute conviction that the body doesn't lie; in fact, that it is a medium for transformation. She has a profound reverence for the wisdom within us and a fearlessness to act spontaneously in response to it. She is ever encouraging us to experiment with poses and movements and to honor what comes to us through them. I hope that you take what she offers here and use it to create or expand a regular yoga practice. It will serve you remarkably well in your quest for health, happiness, and spiritual growth.

—*Carrie Demers, M.D.*
medical director, Center for Health and Healing
Honesdale, Pennsylvania

acknowledgements

I pay homage to H. H. Sri Swami Sivananda, whose approach to yoga therapy has been my guiding light due to the perennial generosity of Pandit Rajmani Tigunait, Ph.D., spiritual head of the Himalayan Institute. I pay homage to H. H. Sir Krishnamacharya, whose yoga method I have had the great fortune to study from his disciple, Sri Srivatsa Ramaswami.

I would like to express the deepest gratitude to my teachers, some of whom are mentioned here. I thank Pandit Rajmani Tigunait, Ph.D., and Pandit Upadesh, Ph.D., of the Himalayan Institute; Swami Veda Bharat, D.Litt., of the Meditation Center; Aileen Crow, my mentor; Bonnie Bainbridge Cohen, Sandy Jamrog, and the faculty of the School for Body-Mind Centering; Mick Grady, Kevin Hoffman, and Dave Gorman, who were my main Hatha teachers; Sri Srivatsa Ramaswami whose work has influenced me greatly; and Lilias Folan, who I feel embodies the true spirit of yoga. I thank Drs. Arny and Amy Mindell, creators of Process Work; Eva Gholson, Dr. Edric Ferdun, and Dr. Sarah Hilsendager of Temple University; Jacki Hand Vagario, Ed Groff, Jan Pforsich, and Jimmyle Kester of the Laban Institute of Movement Studies.

I thank my colleagues, Professor Laura Brooks Rice of Westminster Choir College of Ryder University; Dr. Brian Logan of Logan Chiropractic; April James of the YWCA Princeton; and Deborah Metzger of the Princeton Center for Yoga and Health, for their encouraging support of the development of my work over the years.

I thank my terrific agent Bob Silverstein and the wonderful people at Prima, especially Denise Sternad and Shawn Vreeland, who are both so extremely kind, intelligent, and positive. I thank Pandit Rajmani Tigunait, Ph.D.; Sheela Porter-Smith R.N., C.R.N.P., C.N.M.; and Carrie Demers, M.D., for shedding the light of their expertise on portions of the text, and Rolf Sovik, Ph.D., for clearing up my confusion with Sanskrit. I thank Chris Schmitt, Sally Jenkins, Steve Adams, Alice Preston, and Barbara Konst for their comments on the manuscript in process.

I thank Roger Hill for his good humor and extraordinary illustrations, Chris Schmitt for his patient digital photography, and Mary Cardinal for all her suggestions and guidance in the process of visually representing the practices.

I thank Tony Vlahovic, president of Momentum Fitness, for offering their elegant studio for photography. I thank the models who patiently posed for illustrations: Susan Anderson, Heather Bay, Lenore Denchak, Bonnie Draina, Selene Kaye, Jane Miller, Alice Preston, Esther Rose, Beth Shen, Lise Thompson Brander, and Diane Winstead (with Zachary Aiden Winstead—she had a boy!). I thank Boz Swope for her insightful photography and Lise Thompson Brander for her generous assistance.

I thank each person who has walked into my class or worked with me privately, for you have taught me more about yoga than anyone. I thank my family and friends—Trishia D'Angelo, Charles and Jane Stover, Bal Krishna, Claire Schmitt, Brooke Edwards, Lixian Sun, Marilyn Besner, and Petroska Trosh—for lovingly entertaining my children while I typed. This book would certainly not have been possible without you! I thank Genevieve, Tara, Chris, and Robin for their constant encouragement and support. Finally I thank my parents, Charles and Jane Stover, for demonstrating to me that Love is the Teacher.

every woman's yoga

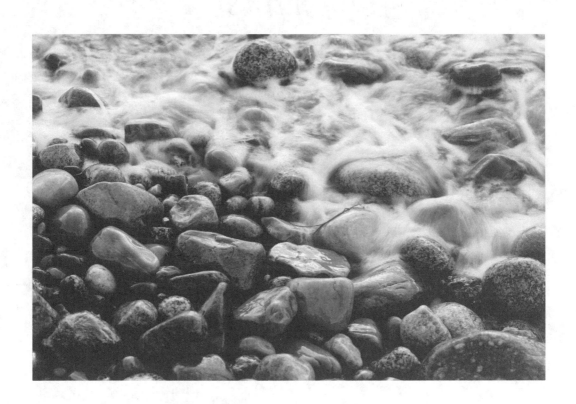

part one

every woman:
body and soul

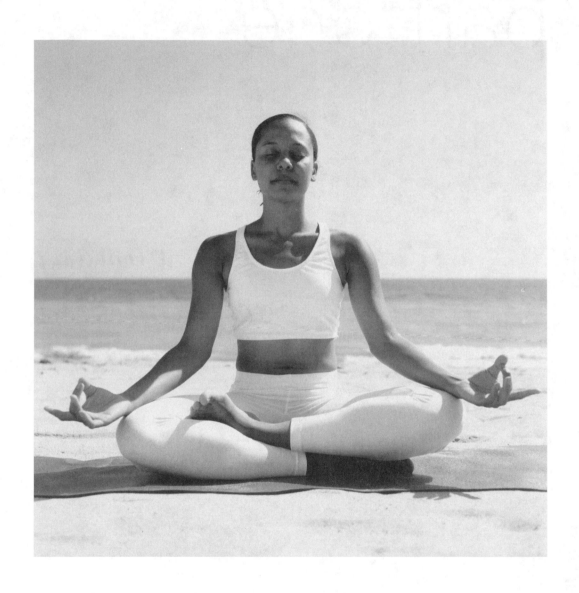

chapter 1

yoga can be your lifeline

The practice of yoga is the endeavor of becoming established in the state of freedom.
—Yoga Sutras of Patanjali, 1.13

Yoga is the master key which opens any lock.
—Sri Swami Satchitananda

Women come to yoga for many different reasons: to keep their bodies strong and supple, look young and feel great, prepare for childbirth, find relief for a specific complaint like back pain, reduce stress, or find support for the transition into menopause. Some are motivated by a vague sense of longing not fulfilled through daily activities. They come lacking deep connection to a purpose, devoid of spontaneity, feeling deadened and out of balance. Each one finds what she is looking for and much more. Vast and inclusive, yoga truly is for every woman. There are many expressions of yoga offering great variety to suit individual needs. The trick is selecting what works for you so you can create a personal practice to meet your needs as they change over the course of your life. This book gives you lots of options so you can choose which practices and approaches to yoga are best for you now and in the future.

yoga science

Yoga is a systematic science, the origin of which reaches back into antiquity. Of the seven schools of Indian philosophy, the Sankhya and Yoga schools share the idea (espoused by the sage Kapila around 600 B.C.) that there are two fundamental aspects of reality. The first is *purusha*, the ancient Sanskrit term for consciousness. The other is *prakriti* or matter. The universe and everything that exists evolved out of the coming together of these two. Odd as this may seem, the postures and practices you see celebrities on TV and models on the covers of magazines demonstrate are based on personal investigation of this notion! This is because yoga is practical and experiential. It provides tangible methods for attaining a state of freedom based in the *Sankhya* philosophy. The central teaching of yoga is that we are always complete, perfect, and Divine. But because we are human, we forget this and instead identify falsely with the body, our personality, our role in life, or other things from the external world. Yoga methods are aimed at redirecting our sense of who we are and, in so doing, our purpose in life.

The word *yoga* comes from Sanskrit, an ancient language whose words often have multiple poetic meanings and innuendos. The most common translation of *yoga* is "union," but it can also mean "discipline," "in conjunction with," and other terms that give slightly different connotations. The verbal root of the word *yoga* is *yuj*, which means "to yoke or harness." A simple way of thinking of yoga is to see it as a way of redirecting our identification from what is impermanent and "yoking" it to our ever-existing universal Self. Yoga's goal is to unite the individual with the Universal; the drop becomes aware that it is the Sea.

many branches, one tree

The term *yoga* is used more or less generically for many different approaches to its universal goal. You might think of yoga as a tree with many branches. The *Bhagavad Gita*, an important classic of ancient India, describes four main branches. However, it is important to note that approaches are not mutually exclusive.

Bhakti Yoga is the path of devotion, faith, and surrender, and is marked by a constant remembrance of or yearning for the Divine. Joan of Arc could have been considered a Bhakti Yogini.

Jnana Yoga is the path of self-inquiry, awareness, and discrimination. It is an intellectually based pursuit of stripping away all false perceptions until the true understanding of one's identity remains. Great Jnana Yogis of late have been Nisargadatta Maharaj and Ramana Maharshi.

Karma Yoga is the path of action, or selfless service in the world. Mother Teresa is considered a great contemporary Karma Yogini.

Ashtanga Yoga, which means eight-limbed yoga, is also called *Raja Yoga*, the royal path. It is the path of yoga systematized by the sage Patanjali in one of yoga's most central texts, the *Yoga Sutras*.

Other traditional paths of yoga exist, such as Tantra Yoga and Mantra Yoga. However, this does not account for the proliferation of names for styles of yoga that have arisen in recent years. Much of what is practiced today in the West stems from what has been handed down over thousands of years through the oral tradition of the teacher–disciple relationship. In many cases, modern schools of yoga have chosen names to distinguish their approach and emphasis from other schools. Even the term *Ashtanga*, the name for the ancient eight-limbed path of Yoga, has come to indicate a specific collection of choreographed Hatha Yoga movements, eye positions, and breathing practices.

The double use of the name has created some confusion. In a few cases, the name given to the type of yoga is merely an individual's name, sort of like Tony's Pizza.

Written roughly two thousand or so years ago, the *Yoga Sutras* are a collection of 196 Sanskrit aphorisms that generally require much explication. Within this text, Patanjali outlines the practices of yoga in eight sections or limbs (hence the name Ashtanga, which means "eight limbed"). This eight-limbed yoga is also termed royal yoga (Raja Yoga) because Patanjali drew on teachings from all the other paths, and because the original Ashtanga Yoga provides a systematic, complete course in self-realization suitable for any sincere aspirant. Raja Yoga works with every aspect of one's physical, mental, and emotional life and does not ask the practitioner to take on any beliefs or deny religious affiliations. Rather, it encourages curiosity, questioning, healthy dis-

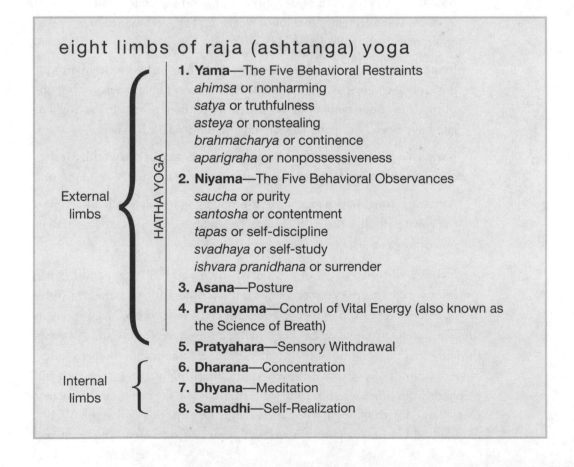

eight limbs of raja (ashtanga) yoga

External limbs

HATHA YOGA

1. **Yama**—The Five Behavioral Restraints
   ahimsa or nonharming
   satya or truthfulness
   asteya or nonstealing
   brahmacharya or continence
   aparigraha or nonpossessiveness
2. **Niyama**—The Five Behavioral Observances
   saucha or purity
   santosha or contentment
   tapas or self-discipline
   svadhaya or self-study
   ishvara pranidhana or surrender
3. **Asana**—Posture
4. **Pranayama**—Control of Vital Energy (also known as the Science of Breath)
5. **Pratyahara**—Sensory Withdrawal

Internal limbs

6. **Dharana**—Concentration
7. **Dhyana**—Meditation
8. **Samadhi**—Self-Realization

crimination, and experimentation and values each person's inner guidance and autonomy. Perhaps this is one reason yoga is so popular in these times of individualism and religious skepticism.

the sun and moon in your practice

I have had the great fortune of studying yoga from two very diverse perspectives. On the one hand, I had the enormous privilege of studying yoga from a master who emphasized its systematic, disciplined, linear progression; he presented yoga from a "masculine" perspective. On the other hand, I also studied yoga within the field of movement under brilliant teachers who valued the unshakable truth found in following the unpredictable and mystifying path of natural curiosity and spontaneity as sensed and expressed through the body in movement—a more intuitive or "feminine" perspective. Over the years, I have come to realize that each approach offsets and complements the other. In this book I try to offer you the best of both but with more detail on the less well-known feminine perspective of yoga. As a result, you have many valid options for creating a yoga practice that fits your body, your needs, and your life today and down the road.

My approach is to honor you as the expert on your self and to encourage you to own that power. People who have been studying a more directive approach than mine sometimes feel frustrated when they first join my class. They expect me to treat them as though they are at a luxurious spa where all their needs are taken care of. But my teachers never taught me like that. They played, they cajoled, they challenged, they prodded, they loved, but they never did it for me. My desire is that you will feel comfortable practicing yoga exactly as you are, with whatever problems you have and whatever hopes you have for overcoming them. If you work honestly and consistently, you will get results. It's a sure thing.

my yoga story

I was introduced to yoga at age five when my mother, for want of a babysitter, began bringing me along to class. We practiced at home with Lilias Folan's extraordinary television series. This delightful time with my mother usually ended in giggles and general horsing around. After a while my mother stopped going to yoga class, but I continued. I can still see the scene: my beautiful teacher, a student of Krishnamurti, and a handful of leotard-clad women, some with beehive hairdos, in the dank cement basement of the YMCA. I practiced at home throughout my school years, disappearing into my room until called for dinner. When my father would come to get me, he'd find me standing on my head or in some other odd position.

When the going got rough in high school, I came home to my yoga-rug-turned-safety-zone to delve into my life force through my breath. I didn't know consciously that I was clearing out the negative feelings from the day or calm-

hatha yoga

Hatha Yoga has enjoyed the place of prominence as the form of yoga best known in the West. Within the framework of Ashtanga Yoga, Hatha Yoga comprises the first four rungs. Traditionally, Hatha Yoga was never seen as a system of mere physical beautification but as a method to purify and fortify the body, breath, and mind, preparing the individual for the meditative pursuit of self-realization. Hatha Yoga harmonizes body, breath, and mind and gives an integrative experience. This is similar to the experience of a performing artist when everything comes together or of an athlete during an exceptional game. Consistent practice brings this integral awareness into everyday life.

Let's look at the various meanings of the Sanskrit word *hatha* as a progression. On a very basic level, *hatha* can be translated as "force." So Hatha Yoga is forceful yoga. From this translation, it is easy to get the impression that in Hatha Yoga you push your body unmercifully into pretzel-like shapes and your only recourse is to dial 911 for help in getting out of the position! Rather, the notion of force here refers to the initial discipline it takes to get out of old habits and into new ones. When you begin to practice, there is bound to be mental, emotional, and physical resistance. In order to continue, it may seem that you have to force yourself to practice. As Swami Veda, a master yogi and Sanskrit expert, explains, "The yogi's body does habitually and naturally what a beginner in Hatha yoga is advised to do by way of an endeavor."

ing and redirecting my mind. I didn't realize then that yoga was saving my life. I just knew at some level that if I stayed close to my breath and kept my body open, I felt fully available to my self. I knew that if I trusted the process, things would move through me and I wouldn't be hurt by them. I knew, even when I was little, that my practice gave me a return to being whole and open. It took me twenty or so years to fully understand that yoga was the rudder that kept me on course through every storm.

I was motivated to write this book after watching a somewhat frail older woman and some overweight red-faced, middle-aged men painfully struggle through a yoga class. The older woman was urged by the gym's membership director to take yoga because it would be good for her arthritic back. I hardly

As the practice of Hatha Yoga becomes familiar, it dawns on you that this forcing is really a dialogue between the exertion of your will and your ability to surrender to what is happening in each moment of your life. The tightrope you walk is learning when and how to apply each one. Now practice involves not only the discipline it takes to organize your life so you can get onto your yoga mat with any regularity (quite a feat in itself!), but it also involves what you do as you work with your body, mind, and emotions, employing your will here, surrendering your efforts or the weight of your body there.

Now you have reached a more refined experience and level of interpretation of the word *hatha*. Of the two words that comprise *hatha*, *ha* means sun and *tha* means moon. This, of course, does not refer to only the external sun and moon in the heavens but to those cosmic forces within us. The sun or *ha* is the more willful, active, assertive, linear, rational, "masculine" aspect of our natural being. The moon or *tha* is the more passive, receptive, nonlinear, process-oriented, intuitive "feminine" dimension of the nature of all things, including us. *Ha* also refers to the passage of breath in the right nostril, and *tha* refers to breath in the left nostril (which you will later read balances active and receptive aspects of our nervous system). At this level of interpretation of the translation, Hatha Yoga expresses the union of two fundamental aspects of nature, the masculine principle and the feminine principle, which are similar to the yin and yang aspects of the Tao. Here yoga as "union" does not refer to a merging that blends away the uniqueness of each original form, but joins *ha* and *tha* together in a marriage of dynamic tension and fruitful attraction.

remembered overhearing this conversation until one day, when I spied this older woman at the back of a very challenging power-type yoga class. A handsome slender young man all of, say, twenty-three and two equally stunning young women were in front performing gymnastic-like poses to music. Their eyes focused on their own images in the mirror or competitively scanned the room for anyone who might challenge their supremacy. They seemed utterly unconcerned with how anyone else in the room was getting along. The older woman and the heavyset grimacing men at the back of the room forced their bodies from one painful failure of a pose to the next.

How do you know when people feel bad about themselves? Is it the look in their eyes, their deflated body positions? Or is it recognizing that feeling in yourself projected into their situation? A sensitive approach to yoga would have been good for this older woman's back, but sadly, after such a failure-based experience, I doubt she will give yoga another try.

yoga's gifts

What yoga has to offer could be a shopping list a mile long. Here are a few of yoga's benefits featured in this book.

OPTIMAL HEALTH

Yoga's health benefits may well be the reason that more than six million Americans, most of them women, now practice yoga. Name a body system, and you will find research that demonstrates yoga's benefit of that system. Through yoga practice, one's cardiovascular and digestive systems are strengthened and cleansed. The immune system is fortified. Every organ and gland is refreshed and gently stimulated. Nerves are toned while the entire nervous system is balanced. The mental chatter of the mind, so powerful in creating or destroying health, is transformed into a one-pointed tool of decisive discrimination.

One student calls yoga her "anti-aging class." She is correct. The Hatha practices give you flexibility, strength, agility, endurance, and balance, which means you have greater ability to move. Our modern world is quickly eliminating natural means for developing and maintaining physical prowess. Children who used to balance on train tracks, jump over streams, and bound through fields of tall grass on their way home now get picked up in car pools. After school they are more likely to play Nintendo than play outside. You may take your ability to move well for granted when you are young, but as your body ages, it stiffens and dries out. Your balance becomes more precarious, you notice more aches and pains, injuries take longer to heal, all of which make you less likely to lead a physically active life. Thus the cycle of debilitation progresses. Hatha Yoga practice doesn't allow this cycle to take hold. Through it you maintain—and quite possibly improve—your ability to move with ease, agility, and power so you can remain active! And because you continue to be active, your body stays healthier.

A fundamental idea in yoga's view of health is that flow is good. Energy, information, nutrients, and wastes all need to move in and out of the body's tissues for vibrant health. Reduce or impair any passageway of flow and you've got a health problem, whether it's emotional buildup related to stress, a sluggish colon, or an artery carrying blood to the brain. Hatha Yoga practice keeps your body's passageways open for business! Your body's areas of stiffness, those places where toxins are stuck, are opened and cleansed, as are your channels of emotional expression and insight.

The baseline of a healthy, mobile, relaxed body means that you will be more comfortable in your skin and therefore less reactive to daily annoyances. The intention of Hatha Yoga is to free you as much as possible from worldly and physical distraction so you can tackle the inner, subtle realms of your mind. Yoga improves your mental acumen, sharpening your mind and prolonging your ability to concentrate. As you learn to willfully and discriminately direct your attention, you reduce the stress caused by your reaction to distraction. Yoga's internal practices help you to clarify your deepest ambitions and connect to your life's purpose. And practice of the *yamas* and *niyamas*, the first two rungs of Ashtanga Yoga, reduces negative indiscriminate actions and negative interactions. Following the *yamas* and *niyamas*—suggestions for making better judgment calls, simplifying your life, and making it more peaceful—is one very practical benefit of Hatha Yoga practice, self-reliance.

SELF-RELIANCE

Yoga encourages sensitivity and intuition. As a woman, you may have been taught that sensitivity is a weakness, a vulnerability to be overcome in a tough world. But yoga practice gives you a context within which to value, even cultivate, your innate intuitive potential. You become better able to locate diminished flow at the various levels of your being—mentally, emotionally, energetically, and physically—before a major imbalance drags you off the playing field. You become better at making choices about what is and isn't good for you. Because of this greater sensitivity, you develop trust in your own inner guidance. As you trust yourself and act spontaneously from your core, you see that the results are worthwhile. This gives you even greater self-confidence and develops self-reliance. You are empowered to transform a habit of negative self-talk into a compassionate outlook, or step back when things aren't going your way to laugh at the dilemma life has provided. When your life is rooted in your own values and purpose, you live fearlessly. Through yoga, you empower yourself to live in harmony with nature and free from self-limitation.

this book and how to use it

This book is divided into four main sections. The first section is introductory. The second section instructs you in basic Hatha Yoga practices. You will find postures that are held, dynamic postures that move with your breathing, longer dynamic sequences sometimes called posture flows, and movement explorations based on the invisible themes that underlie posture practice. This section also includes suggestions for using yoga therapeutically to address concerns most pertinent to women. You will also find a chapter containing breathing practices called *pranayama* that could very well improve your health in dramatic ways. The third section shows you how to use yoga methods for working with your beliefs, thoughts, and emotions. Some books on yoga suggest that practice gives one the ability to gain insight into the generative factors in physical illness. But they don't tell you how this happens or what the yogi does to learn such an important, even life-saving skill. This section does. It gives you two equally valid yet distinct methods for loosening the knots that tie up your life and health. Then a model is outlined to help you work successfully with yourself within the larger spectrum of yoga practice. The final section gives you time-honored guidance about how to get and keep a yoga practice going and suggests lifestyle choices to support your personal goals.

Use this book as a resource to create practices that fit your temperament and lifestyle. After your initial interest has worn off, keep it on a shelf somewhere. Then when you are least in the mood for self-improvement—maybe you're sick, bored, or don't have a magazine—look it over again. I have put enough variety in here so that you'll find something you haven't tried before or a point of view you may not have considered. Perhaps this will renew your interest in what yoga has to offer in every circumstance of your entire life.

This year my youngest student is two and a half years old and my oldest student is eighty-three. I have had the pleasure of exploring individualized practices with people in many states of health and with various concerns, from the challenges of MS and AIDS to a desire for greater ease in lifting a small child or in carrying groceries. I have designed programs to improve the performance of a world-class opera singer, help a plasma physicist "let go" in order to fall asleep, and assist a schoolgirl in developing her pattern of perceptual sequencing. Simply put, yoga works! I am extremely grateful for the presence of yoga in my life and hope you will find it just as valuable. I pass these teachings along to you with that hope in my heart, for yoga truly is the master key to every lock.

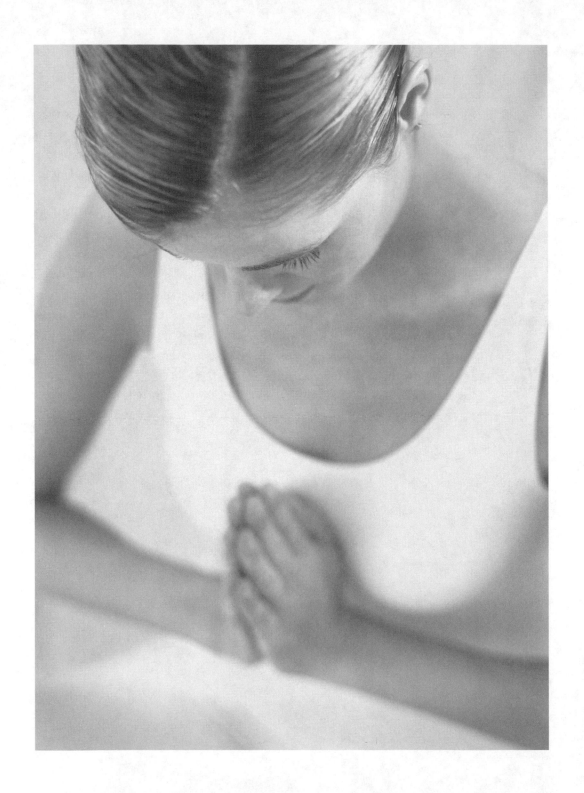

chapter 2

your body is the soul's book

Since man is made in God's image, the body is the soul's book.
—Michelangelo

The body is the soul presented in its richest and most expressive form.
—Thomas Moore

As human beings we are each unique, yet as women we share common challenges of care-giving, balancing work and home life, and feeling good about ourselves in a culture obsessed with youth and beauty. Our bodies change in cycles and over the natural course of time from menarche through menopause, and (if we so choose) through pregnancy, childbirth, and nursing. Our psyches are female; our intelligence is feminine. Even our brains are structured with rich connections to our body wisdom. It is generally agreed that women are more in touch with their bodies and more intuitive than men.

Some approaches to yoga were designed for men who chose monastic life. Superimposing these approaches onto contemporary women's lives is absurd. Women have their periods; run businesses; stay up nights for months with colicky babies; shop and cook for the holidays; care for elderly parents, partners, children, and pets; and may be the hub of a very large family's wheel. Any one woman may be in the midst of all these things at the same time! The approach to yoga practice presented in this book sees these features of a woman's life as a rich context for personal growth, not as demeaning interruptions of the "pure" practice of yoga.

yoga's soul

As Genesis 2:7 states, God formed humankind from the dust of the earth and breathed life into Adam's nostrils. Similarly, the yogic view depicts a consciousness (*purusha*) imbued life force (*prana*) infused into matter, the physical bodies of all living things. *Prana* is the yogic term for the essence of our aliveness, God's breath in the clay of our materially based body. The dust of the earth is *prakriti*, the primal matter out of which everything is formed. So we come into existence, a bolt of consciousness-imbued life force cast into matter—our body. At the same time, a confluence of factors produces a unique swirl of matter's five elements at birth so that each of us begins life's journey with a truly one-of-a-kind constitutional makeup (*dosha*).

This view defines our soul, or *jivan*, as a combination of the pure consciousness at the center of our being with all the personal tendencies and characteristics that distinguish us as individuals. Our soul's expression ought to glow from within our body in each gesture and every action. In our world today, people have little opportunity to move in openly expressive ways. From an early age we are acculturated to conform in behavior and dismiss our need to express our truth in movement. Girls are often taught to limit their "reach" physically and figuratively so as not to appear big, bossy, aggressive, or boyish. We learn that externally defined beauty is a female commodity and are encouraged to manipulate our bodies to conform to these standards. In adulthood the body is treated no better. Both women and men stuff their bodies into synthetic clothes in an effort to create an attractive or powerful image, and run or

the five elements of matter

The Five Great Elements (*Pancha Mahabhuta*) or states of actual physical matter (*tattvas*) emerged from the void. They were ether, air, fire, water, and earth. The first and most subtle of these elements, ether (*akasha*), is not yet material form, but space, the field of distances that separates matter. From ether evolved swirling masses of air (*vayu*), the gaseous state of matter, having the property of mobility or dynamism. These first two elements then combusted into fire (*tejas or agni*), the power of transformation. The residue from this transmutation into fire became the liquid state of matter, water (*apas or jala*), which has the property of flux, or substance without stability. Finally, earth (*pritihivi*), the stable and solid form of matter, resulted from the solidification of all the other elements.

All of creation emerged from a swirling together of these five elements, so that everything in existence is a combination of them. These five elements exist as matter and also as abstract forces. In this worldview, everything that exists out there as real also exists within us in the makeup of our physical bodies and more subtly in the makeup of our character. Do you see from this sense of continuity how yoga's impact on you is comprehensive?

For the sake of expediency, the five elements were combined in theory to form *tridosha*, a fundamental scheme not only for balancing individual health but for viewing balanced health in relation to the worldly environment. *Tridosha* is made up of three principles or forces—*vata, pitta,* and *kapha*—collectively called *doshas*. The more reified elements of ether and air are condensed into one, *vata*, the mobile, less tangible, "spacey" and airy aspect of our humanness. *Vata* is the kinetic principle. The fire element, *pitta*, stands alone as the force of conversion and transformation. It balances the kinetic and potential aspects of our being. The two remaining more substantial elements, water and earth, combine to form the cohesive force *kapha*, the principle of potential energy.

walk on machines to keep their hearts beating and their age from showing. This treatment of our bodies is bereft of soul. Is it any wonder we lose touch with our yearnings and creativity, our natural rhythms, our path in life, and subsequently our health?

yoga's body

The aim of yoga is to recognize our own Divinity and, by adhering to that image, work to untangle this aspect of ourselves from actions that keep us miserable. How is this done? The pathway of Hatha Yoga is through the body. Working with the body's signals, symptoms, and sensations is an especially useful part of this path for women. Deciphering signals becomes soul work when inner sensing and imagination are invited and valued.

As you work your way through the practices in this book, pay close attention to the sensations, images, and impulses that arise. Don't dismiss them as you may be accustomed to doing; they are an important aspect of your inner research (*swadhyaya*). In part three, you will learn to unfold the stories behind these signals. Yoga philosophy offers an integral model of life that explains how yoga works. To show you how completely the mind, emotions, breath, and body are intimately linked in yoga's view of you, two central concepts—the *koshas* and the *chakras*—will be discussed next.

THE *KOSHAS*

The pure consciousness (*purusha*) at the core of our being is often likened to a brilliant light that connects us to all other living beings. It is the individual drop of the vast universal ocean that we are. Because we exist as physical beings, nature has formed subtle to dense layers of matter around this brilliant essence. These layers, called sheaths or *koshas,* can be pictured as fine to dense layers of fabric that conceal the light of pure consciousness.

Picture a light at the center of five concentric circles (see the diagram on the next page). The innermost circle is made of the finest, nearly transparent fabric. This is called the blissful sheath, *ananda maya kosha.* The next layer, slightly opaque, is the intuitive sheath or *vijnana maya kosha.* The next layer, and slightly denser, is the *mano maya kosha* or thinking sheath. These three layers

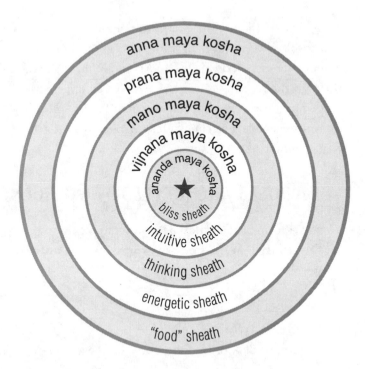

Fig. 2.1. The *Koshas*

make up our "mental" body. It is important to understand that everything that is not pure consciousness is considered "material" in yoga science. So in essence, the mind is a very subtle body. External to the mental layer and denser still is *prana maya kosha,* the energetic sheath or energy body. Acupuncturists work at this level. The external and densest of the five layers is the "food" sheath, *anna maya kosha,* the most tangible aspect of our yoga body.

THE *CHAKRAS:* THE BODY'S CENTERS OF CONSCIOUSNESS

The *koshas* do not function independent of one another but are connected, and more or less coordinated, by centers of energetic awareness called *chakras.* The *chakras* are locations or fields, but not fixed objects by any means. They are whirling confluences of flowing energy and information. In fact, the word *chakra* means wheel or vortex. Each *chakra* acts like a needle that pierces all five layers of being at once. My experience of the *chakras* is that they act like lightning rods, translating the energy and import of experience instantaneously to and through every layer of mind, energy, and physical form. An experience enters awareness at one layer (*kosha*) and infiltrates organically to all the others through the *chakras*. This is how worry can appear as a skin rash, or ambivalence about bearing children can manifest as infertility. The *koshas* and the *chakras* are simple, extremely clear maps to the interrelatedness of psyche and soma (mind and body).

YOGA POSES: ARCHETYPES OF EXPERIENCE

Yoga is a form of self-study best understood through experience. It is based on the reality that the body is expressive. We notice how people are feel-

the seven main *chakras*

Of the many vortices of energy in the body, the seven most prominent are *muladhara, svadhisthana, manipura, anahata, vishuddha, ajna,* and *sahasrara.* Each has a distinct motif that sets the tone of our interactions with the world. The *chakras* illustrate the truly "whole"-istic point of view of yoga, because every aspect of one's being can be studied through them: mental habits, personality, health concerns, postural support, energetic imbalances, and so on. As well as being located in specific areas of the body, the *chakras* are associated with the five great elements bringing the cosmology of the body to a more prominent integration with all of existence.

The *chakras* are aligned along an energy axis that corresponds to our physical spinal column.

1. Muladhara. The first, or root, *chakra,* located at the lowest part of the spine, involves the glandular function of the adrenals and coccygeal body and the coccygeal nerve plexus. *Muladhara* is associated with the earth element. Issues associated with the root *chakra* have to do with instinctual survival. Panic, fear, aggression, and concerns for self-preservation show first-*chakra* involvement.

2. Svadhisthana. In the sacral region, the second center of consciousness, *svadhisthana* involves the sacral nerve plexus and reproductive glands. It relates to the water element and focuses experience on sexuality, sensory pleasure, and survival of the species.

ing through their posture and gestures; they look sad when they move slowly, or a spring in their step says they feel great. In the same way, moving your own body in specific ways, putting it into certain positions, affects your emotions and frame of mind. Postures give us experiences of different points of view and emotions, such as confidence, humility, fearlessness, surrender, and equilibrium. They are like maps, or archetypes of experience, that we can journey through into our primordial relation with all life-forms.

In addition, the postures can be considered metaphors for broader themes in life. We may be stiff or flexible in our mental attitudes, just as we are stiff or flexible in our spine. Posture practice provides direct experience of life prin-

3. *Manipura.* The third *chakra* at the navel region is associated with the solar plexus and the glandular function of the pancreas. It corresponds to the fire element. Issues of domination, sublimation, and the ego involve this *chakra.*

4. *Anahata.* The fourth center, corresponding to the element of air, lies at the level of the heart. It involves the cardiac and pulmonary plexuses, and the thymus gland. The complexity and joy of love and compassion are its domain.

5. *Vishuddha.* The fifth *chakra,* located at the base of the throat, involves the thyroid and parathyroid glands and the pharyngeal plexus. It relates to the ether or space element and involves creativity, expression, and trust in receiving nurturance.

6. *Ajna.* The sixth center, located slightly above the point between the eyebrows, corresponds to the carotid plexus and brain and also involves the pineal gland. *Ajna* relates to the element of the mind, which may not seem like an element of matter at all. From yoga's point of view, however, everything that is not pure consciousness *is* matter, even the very fine vibrations of the activities of the mind. This *chakra* involves introspection, intuition, and seeing the "light" within.

7. *Sahasrara.* The seventh *chakra* sits at the very top of the skull, where a baby's fontanel is located. At the crown of the head, *sahasrara chakra* relates elementally to the Reality beyond form and the experience of vast limitless awareness.

The higher *chakras* have to do with higher states of consciousness and so relate to the innermost sheaths. The lower *chakras,* concerned with the more instinctual aspects of life, relate to the outermost sheaths.

ciples. While doing them, you feel what it is like to bend and what it is like to stand your ground—literally!

learning to read

Asclepius was the ancient Greek god of medicine. Sick people would travel to his temples to be cured. Once there, and after some preparation, a patient would lie down to sleep. It was believed that the treatment for the disease would be revealed through the patient's dream, which the priests would copy down and interpret. My introduction to this Greek god was through a bas-relief in which a serpent was being held by several men over a man's sleeping body. It looked as though the snake was coming out of the sleeping man's ear. The caption explained that the serpent was the man's dream figure, coming from his dreaming body to cure his illness. What resonated so strongly in me was that the image came *from* his body. It was not given to him by an external authority. It wasn't from an insurance company's statistical study or a drug company's list of applications.

The imbalance itself holds the information for its cure. What is needed is to pay attention to the mythology of the signal from within. These days more than a few body workers, psychotherapists, and of late medical doctors have adopted the perspective that the body and mind, psyche and soma (or whatever terms you use) are two sides of the same coin.

Yoga provides an integrated picture of life as a meaningful whole, with each human being living as a unique miniature universe enfolded within the grand process shared by all. By simply focusing awareness on any area of the body, you can learn a great deal about yourself, your energy, your relationship to others and the world, and your issues in this lifetime. By "dreaming in movement" from this area of focused sensitivity, you can learn even more.

Have you ever played the game Battleship, in which you guess the hidden coordinates of an opponent's ship? Outlining a pattern of disharmony and rooting out its cause can be like this game. Disease complexes spread through the *koshas* and often relate to a particular *chakra*. Like a detective, you can trace the pattern of expression of disease or imbalance that manifests in the body, in relationships, in thinking processes, emotions, and energy fluctuations. In your yoga practice, you can enter into your own universe from any point of departure—physical, emotional, mental, intuitive, and so on. Attend to your experience and you are there. Then explore what's up for you today.

With practice, you may at times be able to locate the onset of a state of imbalance, interpret its reason for being there, and learn from yourself what to do about it. This is not New Age mumbo-jumbo or wishful thinking. It is simply a skill developed through the systematic practice of the ancient teachings of yoga science. The practices fortify you for the insights so you are able to address, integrate, and move through issues that might have reduced you to ashes before you began yoga practice. Participating in this process with respect and sensitivity reveals to your conscious mind your own absolutely unique way of functioning in the world.

part two

the vocabulary of yoga practice

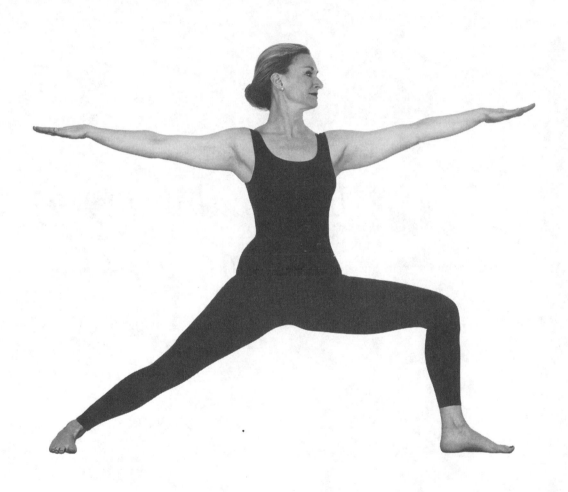

chapter 3

the essential postures for women I
pelvic centering, whole body integration, and balance poses

The power of concentration and imagination applied to the asanas and what they imply puts the body into a kind of "listening mode." Receptivity overcomes the argumentative mode and makes the body relaxed and receptive to its own messages . . .

—Swami Sivananda Radha

Initiation into their own individuality comes for most women through their body.

—Marion Woodman

When you have a dinner party, you get everything ready beforehand in order to relax and enjoy some time with your guests. And because you enjoyed the event, you're more likely to do it again. Preparation is the key to a successful dinner party, and the same is true for a successful yoga practice.

getting started

The following are some tips to help you prepare:

✳ *Find a clean, well-ventilated, quiet place* with enough space to spread out on the floor. Have an area of open wall space and a simple chair nearby to adapt some poses. If you don't have much space, use a closed door as your wall space. Designate this as your yoga space, even if it's only special while you practice. My mat does this for me. When that mat hits the floor, the room I'm in becomes my personal yoga studio, even if it's a moldy old hotel room in India! You may want to light a candle or, if you have space, put pictures up that support what you're doing. Personal touches, no matter how small, make it easier to practice day in and day out.

✳ *The floor surface you'll practice on should be firm enough to balance on one foot,* yet soft enough to lie on comfortably. Use a carpet, a yoga "sticky" mat, or a thin pad; experiment with what works best. One student uses a futon mat on the floor for reclined poses and works on her wood floor for standing ones.

✳ *Go natural with clothing.* Wear nonbinding clothes, preferably made of natural fibers to let your skin breathe. There are lots of great yoga clothes on the market, but sweat pants and a T-shirt work just as well. Check the labels and get ones with a high cotton content because you'll be more comfortable, and toxins that leave you through sweat won't be held against your skin and reabsorbed.

✳ *Because yoga works with your internal organs, you'll need at least two hours of time before you practice after a light meal* and four hours after a heavy one.

✴ *You don't need much stuff to do yoga, but occasionally, props are quite useful.* Places to buy them through mail order are given in appendix D. Household objects work well if you don't want to purchase them. Choose from the following items:

- One or more heavy blankets to fold for supported postures and to cover up for relaxation (I put one over me for seated forward bends on cold winter mornings)

- A strap, rope, belt, or bandanna can extend your limbs when they don't reach far enough

- Two blocks (approximately 9 × 6 × 4) to bring you closer to the floor.

- A firm bolster to support your body in deeply relaxing positions

- A clock

✴ *The ideal time to practice is whenever you can meet the empty stomach requirement!* Classically, the best times are early in the morning before breakfast, just prior to dinner (which works if you aren't the one cooking or if you can prepare dinner ahead of time), and one hour before bed, if you're selecting a less enlivening practice. If you get too pumped at night by your practice, it may disrupt your ability to fall asleep.

✴ *How often? Regularity is key!* It's better to try for short practices three or more times a week than one long one once in a while. One possibility is to schedule a few short practice sessions, say, fifteen minutes, on weekdays, and then give yourself time to indulge in a longer session of ninety minutes to two hours on the weekend. Once you create a regular habit of practice, you can extend the time of your weekday sessions. Once you catch on to how great you feel from your practice, you'll *want to* be on your mat longer and longer. Schedule practice into your day. Make it a priority.

✴ *Yoga in groups.* A weekly class gives you a lot of support, especially when you are just starting out. Search until you find the class that is right for you. Going to class should feel like something you want to do, not something dreadful to endure. A yoga retreat or workshop is another great way to boost your desire and interest in practice. Remembering what it felt like to be there can help you get out of bed and onto your mat when you get home.

what to think when you practice yoga

Believe it or not, all the postures in this book are not as important as the suggestions in this chapter! How you approach your own yoga practice is the true "yoga" of yoga. It's the head game that makes all the difference. You may see blithe young people doing fantastically impossible poses, yet they may be tormented inside. What will help you the most, what yoga has to give that is most important, is the training it gives your mind. The physical training is pretty fabulous, too!

SELF-ACCEPTANCE

You know that the poses unravel the knots in your body, but do you know they have the same subtle and oh-so-potent effect on your mind? Support the inevitable with an attitude of self-acceptance. Put the critics outside your practice room. Gag the judge. Do whatever it takes to make your yoga practice time a safe, dare I say sacred, place for you. Cultivate unconditional acceptance of yourself in exactly this moment. This now is the practice of yoga (*atha yoganushasanam*).

It's funny, but once you get even a little of this acceptance thing going, your progress soars. But if you fake it to make your progress soar, then it won't. Take this attitude of acceptance along to your class or workshop so you won't get swept up into anyone else's competitive head trip.

GET INTO IT

Focus inward and listen to what's there. You may have learned to do just the opposite. You may know very well how to get through something by turning off the sensations from the body and the responses from within. Many of us have approached fitness training with a "no pain, no gain" philosophy. With this point of view, we may be able to get by for some time, but as the body ages, our weakest link—whether it is a knee, a hamstring, or the low back—is bound to give. Yoga practice unravels these tendencies to deny parts

from doing to being

Attention on the breath is an instantaneous way to draw the attention inward. When you focus your attention on feeling your body breathe, you switch instantly from doing to sensing in the present moment.

of ourselves. Through it we release tensions that have accumulated, cleanse, and actually make better progress.

Yoga trains us to work intensely and with great concentration, listening attentively to the feedback from our body so we become even more responsive beings. As we refine our attention to the body's sensations in practice, we find we have opened the door to a world of infinite interest and fascinating self-discovery.

TAKE THE JOURNEY

Each pose is a form that creates a pattern of energetic flow in your body. In fact, any ordinary position, such as sitting at a desk, will cause energy to flow in a certain way. In yoga practice, we capitalize on this principle by expanding the body into special forms. Then we breathe, sometimes in special ways, so as to run energy that nurtures, cleanses, and otherwise supports life. Postures show us where we have greater or lesser flow. A stiff area means little flow. Focus on identifying these spots (some cry out and need no search party, others are much more subtle!), then be present with them once you do. As you pay close attention to how these areas feel, the body will teach you how to move and what to do to release the stiffness.

Sometimes a cigar is a cigar. Your calves are tight because you ran in the cold wind in shorts yesterday. Other times, as you attend to the areas of tension in a pose, something else makes itself apparent. You may notice an emotion that was not there before or a memory of some event. You may catch a glimpse of something you've forgotten. These perceptions, fleeting or recurrent, are easy to dismiss. Yet they can lead you down a fascinating avenue of practice. These ephemeral perceptions take you into the language of your soul. The body is always speaking the language of true feelings. Why else do we blush when we don't want to? As you refine inner listening skills during yoga practice, you will be able to follow the wild currents of expression always present in the body's mind.

MIND THE EDGE

Here's a common setup for disaster. You see a perfected posture in a book or on a yogini in the front of class. You get the image in your mind and decide, without consulting your body, that this will work for you. You slam-dunk the pose and find yourself out for two months with a pulled or torn muscle. Don't do it!

Instead, focus on what you're feeling. You definitely want to feel the stretch, intensely if you're up to it, but not pain. Pain makes you want to get out of there fast. Pain sets up conflict inside of you: Part of you demands you stay; another part (such as your screaming hamstring muscles) wants you to stop. This is no longer yoga practice. You're practicing yoga when you explore your interest in and capacity for heading toward the limit of a stretch. Maybe the maximum physical limit is right for you, or maybe you want to hang back. Perhaps you're most interested in learning to work very gently with your body.

The yoga postures are ancient forms of archetypal experience. They are based in our human anatomy and in our evolutionary history. They take us to our physical limits and at the same time open us to the terrain of our psyche. Both of these aspects of our total being are stretched in yoga practice.

In both these dimensions, we may reach the limit of our comfort. These limits are literally and figuratively our edge. It's important to approach practice by being mindful of these edges each day. They shift like the tides. One day you may feel as though you want to open all the stops in your life and sweep your body and mind clean. Another day you may feel weak, tired, and vulnerable. Respect your edges. If you use force, you won't expand your edges; they'll snap back tighter. Or worse, you'll plunge over them into injury or emotional upheaval.

Another setup for backlash is to allow someone else to coax you into going more deeply into a posture than you are mentally or emotionally ready for. One form of yoga therapy instructs that all tension is bad and should be eradicated. The therapist physically presses the practitioner into a position the body could not get into by itself. People often feel psychologically beat up from a session like this. Edges are there for good reason; they serve a purpose. Honor this.

Still another ill-fated way to deal with edges is to not deal with them at all. A competitive sprinter once took my class. She was impatient with the slowness of the stretches and with how stiff she was. It seemed hard on her ego to know that women who could easily be her mother were "better than her" at stretching. She switched to a style of yoga that emphasized strength. Later I heard that she injured the tendons in her ankle and was out of competition. She probably thought yoga was no good and couldn't help her.

MENTAL METTLE

Yoga practice is a powerful way to work with your mind. Through it you can study your current mental and emotional habits while cultivating ones that support who you are and where you want to go in life. There is a repetitive prayer (*mantra*) in the yoga tradition that uses the image of a vine growing into a thorny tangled patch. The vine asks the Divine to help it disentangle itself from this troublesome direction and thread it instead around a nearby straight and life-giving stalk. Yoga practice helps us observe our thought patterns. We can then decide which ones are not useful and which ones are worth cultivating.

When you get into a posture, particularly a challenging one, observe your thoughts. What do you say to yourself? What happens? Do you push your body and tune out your sensations? Does an internal critic step up to the mike? Do you zone out? Are you bored? Many people don't even want to know this much about themselves, so the fact that you are even reading about this process is to be congratulated. Welcome to the path!

At this point, yoga directs us not to go crazy about our mental game. It instructs us to sit back and watch the mind run its program. It's sort of like when you mistakenly hit the play button on your VCR. You're just playing a tape, reacting rather than responding. From the cool observer's point of view, you have a chance to choose your response. The better you get at stepping back and watching the mind show, the more decisively clear and peaceful your life will be.

your yoga user's guide

As you begin practicing the poses described in chapters 3, 4, and 5, keep these general thoughts in mind:

✳ *The first version of each pose I describe is of average difficulty.* Most adults in my beginning classes are able to do the pose straight away or with some slight adaptation. You'll see "Make It Easier" and "Challenge Me" under the description of most poses to give you more options for tailoring your practice.

✳ *For every tip or idea I have included, there were at least ten more tips I could have added* that didn't make it onto the page. This is your yoga practice, and you are in charge, so feel free to adapt the postures as needed and improvise new variations. Be creative! I trust you'll use common sense. Seek out a qualified yoga teacher for assistance if needed. When you get into a pose, noodle around. Have you ever seen first graders eat lunch? Not one of them sits still. They are constantly in motion. Resist making tombs of the poses. Keep sensing how your body fits into them through little movements here and there. Adjust. Then adjust again and again! I don't say this throughout, but this is a very important way to own your practice.

✳ *My mission is to put you in the driver's seat of your own yoga practice as soon as possible.* The poses are grouped into categories, so you can select ones that are perfect for you in designing your own balanced practice. Yes, there are guidelines. Yes, I have sample practice routines. But more than anything else, I want to hand you the keys so that the postures described here jump out of this book and into the rest of your life.

✳ *It helps to visualize a pose before you do it,* especially if you've never done it before. This helps your nervous system plan ahead.

✳ *I don't say this every time (yawn), but move into and out of every pose slowly.*

✳ *Sometimes I'll ask you to hold a posture, classically called an* asana. Get into the position with good body alignment and support and feel just the right amount of stretch or work. Make any adjustments you need and then hold the pose. Stay alert to the body's sensations to determine when to come out. I may ask you to stay there for three breaths, but override me as needed. Stay for less, or stay for more. I'm just the tour guide.

✳ *If getting down on the floor is difficult, do the practices on a firm sofa or bed.* One of my senior clients has a guest room with a fold-out futon sofa in it. Now that she practices yoga, she keeps the futon bed out and does her sitting and lying practices on top of it.

✻ Other practices described are moving sequences, called *vinyasa krama*. I'll ask you to move into or out of a position in a specific way. Or you'll use movement to connect two or more postures together in a loop. This is like when you're washing a window. You have the standing and washing position, you have the bending-over-the-bucket position, and you have the movement in between that gets you back and forth.

✻ Whenever you remember, breathe fully, focusing on the movement of the diaphragm, which is at the bottom of the rib cage. It's like a horizontal dome that lowers to flatten when you breathe in and rises back up when you breathe out. (There's more on this in the breathing section.) When you breathe fully, you may notice the breath slows down. This is a good thing. Slow the breath by allowing it to be fuller longer, but not by tensing up and making more resistance for the air.

the essential posture practices

Of course, men do these yoga practices, too, but I've compiled this selection and approach specifically to meet the needs of women, with variations for all ages and abilities. This Vocabulary of Yoga Practice section contains all the practices to choose from in designing your personal practice. This chapter and chapters 4 and 5 contain the classical poses, chapter 6 provides approaches to dynamic movement practices, and chapter 7 describes powerful yet subtle vitality-promoting techniques, known as *pranayama*. Chapter 8 offers specific practice selections for special times and health needs. The final section of the book helps you to put it all together to create a personal practice that perfectly suits you and your lifestyle.

POSTURE: STEADINESS AND COMFORT

I've provided several versions of most poses, so you can keep track of which versions are right for you as you explore the practices. You may also want to reflect on the categories of practice. What are you most interested in?

Strength? Toning? Stress reduction? You might choose the entire first category, Pelvic Center Poses, as the heart of your practice for a Pilates-like core-strengthening routine. Each category is laid out sequentially, so you could do all the poses in one category in order if you wish.

Nine categories of practice are outlined below. They include postures focused on (1) the pelvic center, (2) whole body integration, (3) balance, (4) side bending, (5) shoulder mobility and back bending, (6) twisting, (7) hip mobility and forward bending, (8) inversions, and (9) relaxation. Use this section as a reference to learn each posture you are interested in. Then go to chapter 7 when you are ready to put them together with other yoga practices to design your personal plan.

Category 1. Pelvic Center Poses

After twenty-seven years in the fitness industry, I've yet to meet a woman who wants the upper body of Mr. T. Yet many yoga programs based on male anatomy emphasize upper body development. In general, men have broader shoulders, larger chests, and longer arms, giving them the mechanical advantage in performing challenging upper body postures. Some women do rise to the challenge, albeit with more difficulty. Ginger Rogers did every dance step with Fred Astaire—in high heels and backwards!

Most women want to focus on their pelvic region, abdomen, hips, thighs, and buttocks. Our female anatomy, coupled with the effects of childbearing on pelvic muscle tone and fat accumulation, makes this the area of concern for most. I call this area the pelvic center. Progress in any fitness regimen, including Hatha Yoga, relies on strength in this central area. In fact, strength in the pelvic center is a marker of good health, vital reserve, and longevity. A yoga routine that focuses on the pelvic center will give you strong, flexible muscles and an ability to move powerfully with balance and grace. Why? Because you're not bulking up as in classic weight training, which stiffens isolated muscles as they enlarge. You're working with integrated whole body coordination, training your nervous system to be more skillfully responsive while you lengthen muscles as you strengthen them, like dancers. Naturally, you become more graceful, agile, quicker, and stronger, which is why many athletes seek yoga training to enhance their performance.

This section begins with the internal strengthening practices that are essential to core strength in every activity, from carrying groceries to finishing

gentle limbering practices and warm-up

Depending on a number of factors (time of day and season, your age, physical condition, time and practice choices), you may need to loosen up first. This easy warm-up can be done standing. It serves as a remedial practice for people who are not at the moment capable of doing the classical poses and can be used as a break from tedious sedentary work at the office, for example:

- Circle your wrists and ankles in both directions.
- Stretch your arms overhead, then lower them; repeat two or more times. Try different pathways up and down.
- Clasp your hands, palms together, overhead, and draw an imaginary circle on the ceiling. For more work, make the circle larger and larger. Go both directions three or more times.
- Swing your arms across-open and up-down and on diagonals many times.
- Circle your arms at your shoulders three or more times, and make figure eights.
- Roll your shoulders forward and back three or more times, together and alternately.
- March in place, lifting your knees and arms high.
- Circle your thigh in the hip joint, standing on one leg at a time. Or standing wide, roll your hips in a large, even circle each way several times.
- Chop. Clasp the arms overhead, breathe in, and look up. Bend your knees, exhale, and bend forward to chop between your legs.
- Twist to each side. Turn your head, reach your arms around behind you, and allow your trailing heel to come off the floor. Alternate several times.
- Cat Stretch (*Bidalasana*). Bend your knees; place your hands on them. Exhale, curl your spine, inhale, arch your spine. Generally move your spine all around; get the kinks out. You can also do this on your hands and knees.
- Hang over. Bend your knees and let your spine fold over from your hips. Let your head and arms dangle. If this is too much stretch, place your hands or elbows on your knees or thighs. Breathe and relax here. Roll slowly up.

the center of health

The rolling and squeezing actions of pelvic center practices massage your internal organs, which keeps them healthy. Fresh blood moves through them, their tissues are toned, and they are stimulated and cleansed by these motions. Even if you work out in conventional Western ways, add some Hatha Yoga to your regimen. Remember, your biceps don't keep you alive, but your internal organs sure do!

a triathlon. The control of these muscles is learned in some martial arts and dance forms, but their isolation as an exercise is unique to yoga. Yoga routines that include core support through the pelvic center give you the edge in all movement forms and exercise regimens. They form the basis for integral strength throughout the pelvic center and the entire body and are of special importance to women who plan to have or have had children.

ROOT LOCK (*Mula Bandha*)

THE POWER OF THE POSE: Strengthens pelvic floor muscles, stimulates and tones pelvic nerves, tones the urogenital system, benefits peristalsis (elimination).

Sit in an erect position on the floor or in a chair with a firm seat. Sense the canoe-shaped area of your perineum. Slowly squeeze this area toward the central point (the center of your perineal body), drawing it up slightly, and then slowly release. It's like the seat in the middle of the canoe. If you have trouble moving this area, roll up a sock and place it just behind the vaginal opening. Repeat this exercise ten to twenty-five times. Try to isolate only these muscles and keep your abdominal and buttocks muscles relaxed. Be patient! If this is easy for you, go on to the next variation.

Begin by contracting as in the previous exercise, shortening the muscles of your pelvic floor toward a central point just behind your vaginal opening. Hold that contraction while narrowing your vaginal barrel by contracting its muscles. Release your vaginal barrel; then release your pelvic floor muscles.

Now try this Root Lock in coordination with your breath.

As you slowly exhale:

Contract your pelvic floor to the center point (the center of the canoe seat).

Lift your pelvic floor and tighten your lowest section of your vaginal barrel.

Continue to lift and tighten your middle section.

Maintain the lift of the pelvis floor as you tighten the upper portion.

As you slowly inhale:

Release the upper portion.

Release the middle portion.

Release the lower portion and pelvic floor.

Begin with ten repetitions and work up to twenty-five, adding in increments of five.

ABDOMINAL LIFT (*Uddiyana Bandha*)

THE POWER OF THE POSE: Strengthens abdominal muscles, massages abdominal and pelvic organs, improves circulation and nerve function throughout the torso, improves digestion and elimination, helps regulate adrenal glands, and helps redistribute abdominal fat. Same position as Solar Energizer.

advanced practice alert!

At Spanda (my yoga movement therapy practice) we have been experimenting for several decades with breath coordination while articulating the muscles of the pelvic floor and surrounding area. We have found that breathing out as you contract your muscles is the best pattern to strengthen the pelvic floor, especially for beginners. We advise advanced female students who are able to work with other breath patterns in this practice to include this supportive version in their daily routine. Some teachers teach an opposite breathing pattern—breathing in on contraction and out on release. We feel this version is more demanding, as it challenges the strength of the pelvic floor muscles. It may be beneficial after all these muscles are sufficiently strong and flexible and you are able to isolate contractions in the different sections of your pelvic floor and vaginal barrel. However, to do this before you have gained sufficient strength and subtle awareness will be detrimental to your progress.

Caution: Do not do the Abdominal Lift when pregnant or have colitis, intestinal ulcer, hiatal hernia, unmedicated high blood pressure, glaucoma, raised intercranial pressure, or overactive thyroid.

Stand with your feet slightly wider than your hips. Keeping your spine straight, lean forward to place your hands on your thighs just above slightly bent knees. Exhale as fully as possible, and then tuck your chin into the hollow of your throat. Without inhaling, draw your abdomen up and back toward your spine. Hold to your comfortable capacity. To release, first lift your head to level, then relax your abdominal muscles. Repeat six to ten times.

MAKE IT EASIER: Do the practice sitting in a chair. Remember, while you breathe out, draw your abdomen in. It's the same movement as when you cough or shout. As you breathe in, release.

SOLAR ENERGIZER (*Agni Sara*)

THE POWER OF THE POSE: Strengthens abdominal muscles, massages abdominal and pelvic organs, improves circulation and nerve function throughout the torso, improves digestion and elimination, helps regulate adrenal glands, and helps redistribute abdominal fat. Stimulates dormant energy and improves overall health.

In this practice, you coordinate the contractions of both your pelvic floor and your abdominal wall with your breath. This may seem complicated at first, but it is such a powerful vital practice that it is definitely worth learning!

Stand with your feet slightly wider than your hips. Keep your spine straight. Lean forward to place your hands on your thighs just above slightly bent knees. Draw upward sequentially from your pelvic floor to your stomach,

Caution: Do not do the Solar Energizer when pregnant or have colitis, intestinal ulcer, hiatal hernia, unmedicated high blood pressure, glaucoma, raised intercranial pressure, or overactive thyroid.

bottom to top, as you breathe out. Then release the contraction sequentially from top to bottom as you breathe in. The image I use to help this coordination is an elevator in a three-story building. The people get in on the ground floor and ride the elevator up to the third floor. Then they come all the way down—third floor, second floor, first floor—to get out on the ground floor.

Slowly exhale:

Squeeze your pelvic floor and lift its hammock-like webbing.

Continue the contraction through your vaginal barrel from the bottom to the top.

Retaining these contractions, pull your abdominal wall back in a rolling motion from its lower portion to its higher portion.

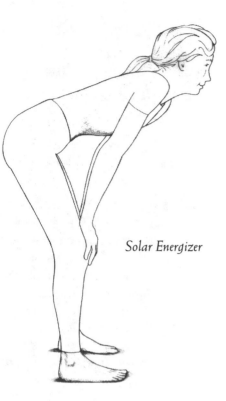

Solar Energizer

not all crunches are created equal

Most women want to elongate and narrow their torso with abdominal exercise. *Agni Sara* is the perfect exercise for this, as it tones all the abdominal muscles, not just the *rectus abdominus,* which are targeted in typical sit-ups. Sit-ups done without awareness of the function of the abdominal wall muscles can actually compress and thicken the abdomen.

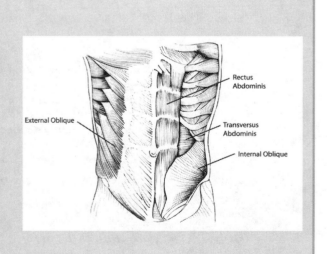

External Oblique

Rectus Abdominis

Transversus Abdominis

Internal Oblique

benefits of solar energizer, *agni sara*

Agni means fire in Sanskrit. Like the sun in the sky, *agni* is the internal furnace of the body, providing heat and the energy of transformation. At the body level, strong *agni* helps us use the nourishment we take in. We need a strong flame to digest our food without residue. Of course, high-quality foods like fresh fruits and vegetables are most easily assimilated, burning clean like any good fuel. When our physical digestion is strong, we feel well after eating and are hungry again in four or so hours.

Agni Sara keeps the digestive fire stoked and stimulates the function of the element of fire in your whole being. This fire gives us strong immunity, as the white blood cells are like white fire in the body, decisively assimilating toxins. This goes for toxic experiences as well. At times when our fire is overwhelmed, we can't assimilate indigestible experiences. The cause could be a single event or daily affronts that have added up. Strong *agni* gives us the power of discrimination, the ability to sort things out. Determination, joy, passion, and courage are all fueled by *agni*. Yoga practices are both physical and metaphysical. This is why the benefits of exercises such as *Agni Sara* are difficult to list. You experience them in your body and in your life at a level of implicit understanding.

If you've got anything left, pull your stomach up under your rib cage. (See why you don't want to eat before you practice?)

Slowly inhale:

Release your stomach and upper portion of your abdominal wall; then allow the relaxation to roll down your abdomen. Let it soften.

Release your vaginal barrel from the top to the bottom.

Finally, release your pelvic floor muscles.

This will take some time to perfect. It requires concentration and subtle articulation. *Agni Sara* can be done while performing certain postures and posture sequences.

DESK POSE (*Dvipada Pitham*)

THE POWER OF THE POSE: Opens chest, stretches front of body, strengthens pelvis and legs, and acts as a gentle inversion.

Desk Pose

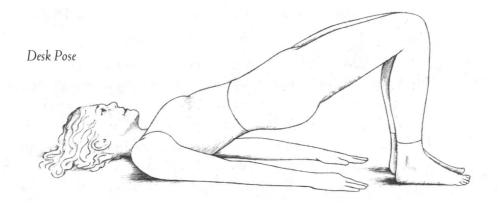

Like all the postures, this one can be done in many ways. A number of features make it important. We'll focus on rolling off the floor from the tailbone and engaging the muscles in the pelvis and backs of the thighs.

To give you a sense of these muscles at work, first try the pose as a movement pattern (*vinyasa krama*). Lie supine with your knees bent, soles of your feet on the floor. Inhale to curl your tailbone up between your legs, then push through your feet to roll your pelvis and low back off the floor. Exhale to roll down, releasing your tailbone as the breath finishes. Repeat several times. Try raising your arms overhead as your torso rises while you inhale, and then returning them to the sides of your body as you exhale.

When ready, roll up as you have just done and hold the posture (*asana*) for three breaths or longer. Feel your feet ground into the floor and the work of the hamstrings and pelvic muscles.

UPWARD-FACING BOAT SERIES (*Navasana*)

THE POWER OF THE POSE: Strengthens abdominal and pelvic muscles, stimulates all body systems, tones organs, and eliminates nervous tension.

I must admit, I'm an abdominal-strength maniac. But washboard abs aren't the only way to be incredibly strong in this area. Here are five suggestions for working with the muscles in the front of the torso and the organs that underlie them. Feel free to improvise with these practices by adding repetitive movements, altering leg positions, or twisting to each side. To do this as a series, do one repetition of each version, that is, one upper, one lower, one full, and so on for as many sets as you can do comfortably.

This pose has many variations. For our purpose, we will break it down into two parts: upper body lifts and lower body lifts.

VERSION 1: Half Upward-Facing Boat Pose (*Ardha Navasana*)—Upper. Focus on using the abdominal muscles while performing the pose. Lie on your back, knees bent, soles of your feet on the floor. Curl your chin to your chest. Exhale; reach your arms toward your knees to lift the upper back and shoulder blades off the floor while pressing your lower back into it. Slowly lower the upper back and shoulders. Five to ten repetitions are a good start. Keeping the lift low will ensure that you are working the abdominal muscles and not just the hip flexor muscles.

A variation that includes a different section of the abdominal wall is to curl up and reach diagonally across the body. Alternate right arm to left knee, left arm to right knee, keeping the chin to the chest. Five to ten repetitions is a good start.

VERSION 2: Half Upward-Facing Boat Pose (*Ardha Navasana*)—Lower. A good test of your progress in strengthening your abdominal muscles is to lift and lower your legs while lying on your back. If your hip-flexing muscles are strong, they'll take over. To ensure you are strengthening the abdominal muscles, you must be able to keep the low back pressed into the floor and the belly from bulging out.

Lie supine with your knees folded into your chest, arms along your sides on the floor. Keeping the leg bent, lower the right foot to the floor and then fold it back in; repeat with the left foot. Remember to keep your back to the floor and your abdomen pulled in. Next, extend each leg to a 45-degree angle off the floor and then draw it back to your chest, bending the knee. Check to make sure you're keeping your lower back flat on the floor. Extend each leg

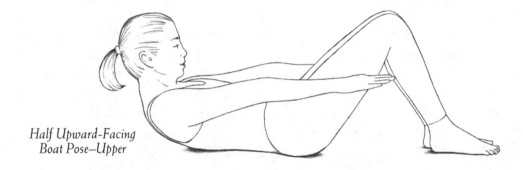

*Half Upward-Facing
Boat Pose—Upper*

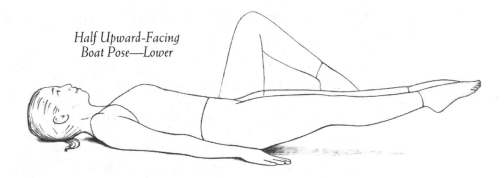

*Half Upward-Facing
Boat Pose—Lower*

and lower it to a few inches above the floor and then draw it back to your chest, bending your knee. When this exercise eventually becomes easy, try it with both legs extending and folding together. You must keep your back flat and your belly in for strengthening. If you can manage to exhale and add a pelvic floor contraction (*mula bandha*) each time you extend one or both legs out, you'll be supporting these strengthening movements internally.

VERSION 3: Full Upward-Facing Boat Pose (*Navasana*). Sit with your legs outstretched in front of you and your back straight. Exhale to tilt back while drawing your knees into your torso. Inhale to extend your legs as you stretch your arms forward, parallel to the floor. Breathe evenly for three breaths or longer. Work toward remaining in the pose comfortably for longer and longer periods of time.

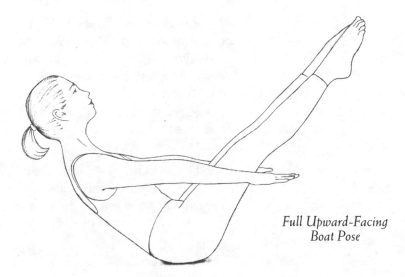

*Full Upward-Facing
Boat Pose*

CHALLENGE ME: Dynamic Upward-Facing Boat Pose 1 (*Navasana Vinyasa Krama 1*)

(Definitely try this one first!)

This practice has four repetitive positions:

1. Begin on your back with arms outstretched overhead. Breathe in.

2. As you exhale, curl your tailbone under, bring your chin to your throat, and roll up, bending your knees. Keep your upper arms near your ears.

3. Inhale to sit tall, reach up, and extend your legs out along the floor (*Dandasana*).

4. Exhale, roll to the back of your pelvis, curling your tailbone under, drawing your abdominals back, chin to chest. Your arms can reach forward if needed. Continue rolling down as you bend your knees. Inhale to stretch your arms overhead and extend your legs once again along the floor.

If you can do version 1 with your abdominals pressed back as you roll up and down, you're ready for this next outrageously strengthening practice!

guiding principle: make friends with the breath

There is a saying in yoga: "The breath is the link between the mind and the body." By focusing on the breath while you practice, you unite these levels of your being. Because of this intimate coupling, working with the breath during yoga practice leads to a powerful integrative experience. An excellent way to check in with your state of being is to observe the flow of breath. What does it feel like? Shallow and quick, long and deep; is it difficult to breathe in or out? What else do you notice? As you repeatedly check in with your breath flow, you'll begin to recognize patterns that tell you more precisely what's up.

Alternatively, you can direct the breath in many different ways. You can stoke it for more power in a challenging posture sequence, or soften it to a delicate long thread in a supported pose. The possibilities are limitless. Explore this sacred link of breath between your body and mind during yoga practice and in your everyday life.

A FURTHER CHALLENGE: Dynamic Upward-Facing Boat Pose 2 (*Navasana Vinyasa Krama 2*)

(The same sequence as above. Just lift your legs off the floor into the Upward-Facing Boat Pose):

1. Begin on your back, with your arms outstretched overhead. Breathe in.

2. As you exhale, curl your tailbone under, bring your chin to your throat, and roll up, arms remaining overhead. Bending your knees, draw your feet off the floor so that you're balancing on the back of your pelvis.

3. Inhale to sit tall, extend the legs to a 45-degree angle off the floor while stretching your arms parallel to the floor along the outsides of the legs. Flatten your back by pushing down on the tailbone.

4. Exhale to roll to the back of your pelvis. Bend your knees to roll all the way down to the floor. Inhale to stretch your arms overhead and extend your legs along the floor. Repeat six to eight or more times to your comfortable capacity.

LOCUST POSE (*Shalabhasana*)

THE POWER OF THE POSE: Strengthens arms, lower back, pelvic and abdominal muscles; stimulates spinal nerves (especially entire sympathetic autonomic nervous system); benefits digestion; relieves abdominal pressure and constipation.

VERSION 1: Half Locust Pose (*Ardha Shalabhasana*). We'll begin with this pose, which is powerful and demanding in itself. You gain all the benefits with this pose. Please don't push yourself to accomplish the full pose if it's not right for you!

Lie prone with your legs together. Place the flat part of your chin (the part you see when you look in the mirror, not the underneath edge) on the floor. Your

> **Caution:** Do not do the Locust Pose if you have back pain and disc injury or you're pregnant.

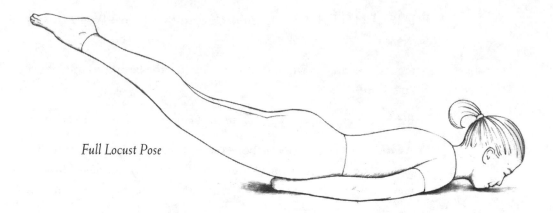

Full Locust Pose

arms are important in this posture. If you've ever hit a volleyball upward with your forearms, you already know the feeling of what to do with your arms in this pose. Place your hands under your groin or upper thighs. Make fists if this doesn't hurt your hands. Exhale and imagine one of your legs growing a little longer as you lengthen it away from your hip along the floor. Inhale and lift your leg up by lengthening it more. Press your forearms into the ground and breathe evenly for three breaths. Exhale as you slowly lower your leg. Repeat the lift with your other leg. As this becomes easy, repeat alternating several times, holding for longer amounts of time.

MAKE IT EASIER: There are two ways to make this pose easier. One is to tuck under the toes of the leg you're not lifting and allow this knee to press into the floor as you lift the other leg. Another way to strengthen the muscles without being on your belly is to get on your hands and knees and straighten one leg out behind you. Be careful to lift from your hip while keeping your back strong and flat (don't let it sag).

VERSION 2: The Full Locust Pose (*Shalabhasana*). This pose requires you to lift both legs. Lie prone with your legs together. Place the flat part of your chin on the floor. Place your hands under your groin or upper thighs. Make fists if this doesn't hurt your hands. Exhale to lengthen both legs away from your torso. Inhale and lift both legs up while pressing your fists into the floor. Breathe evenly for three breaths. Exhale as you slowly lower. As this pose becomes easy, repeat twice more, holding for longer amounts of time.

Caution: In the next three poses, as you bend your knees, be sure to align them over your toes. Keep a perfect footprint of your heel, pad, and all five toes evenly weighted on the floor and pointed forward.

CHAIR POSE (*Utkatasana*)

THE POWER OF THE POSE: Strengthens leg, pelvic, and back muscles; massages heart; and tones abdominal organs.

Stand with your feet close together. Breathe in to lengthen your spine upward and stretch your arms overhead. Keep this lift as best as you can while you breathe out and bend your knees to lower to a half-squat position. Keep your heels on the floor. Make sure your knees go directly over your toes. Breathe fully and softly focus your eyes on something in front of you. Keep your back long and draw your pelvic floor up (*mula bandha*). Stay for three or more breaths. As your legs and pelvis gain strength, you may deepen the position. As you deepen the pose, keep your thighs just above parallel to the floor to protect your knees.

MAKE IT EASIER: Dynamic Chair Pose (*Utkatasana Vinyasa Krama*). Go down into the bent knee position (exhale) and back up (inhale) three or more times as a great way to condition your thigh muscles to be able to hold the pose. Keep those knees over your toes!

CHALLENGE ME: Perform the Chair Pose with Solar Energizer (*Utkatasana* with *Agni Sara*). Keep your back long and your knees over your toes. Exhale to squeeze, inhale to release, several times.

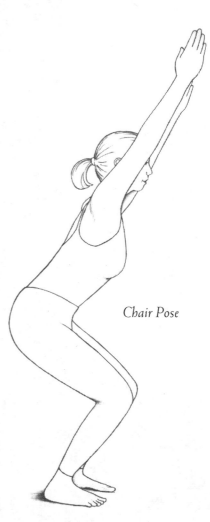

Chair Pose

Caution: Do not do the Powerful Pose during pregnancy or if you have a pro-
lapsed uterus.

POWERFUL POSE (*Ugrasana*)

THE POWER OF THE POSE: Strengthens leg, pelvic, and back muscles;
massages heart; tones the uterus.

Begin this practice as a dynamic pose (*vinyasa krama*). Then, if you feel up to
it, hold the pose at the end. Done this way, you'll warm up your hip joints and
the deep muscles of your pelvis before calling on them to hold the posture.

Stand with your legs wide apart. Rotate your toes out from your hips (like
a dancer's second position). Breathe in to stretch upward throughout your entire torso while stretching your arms overhead. Breathe out, slowly bend your
knees, aiming them diagonally out to the sides over your toes. Open your arms
to the sides at shoulder height. As you do this, feel your legs rotate outward

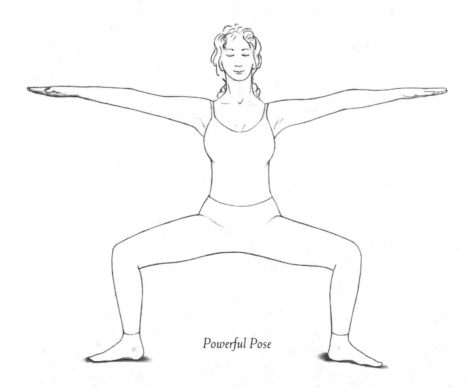

Powerful Pose

from your pelvis. Breathe in and slowly come up once again, stretching your arms overhead. Repeat three or more times. Are you interested in using *Agni Sara* to work deeply with your abdominal muscles and pelvic floor as you lower and lift into this posture? Try it.

Now lower as above and hold the pose to your comfortable capacity. Breathe deeply. Feel the vital surge in this pose. Wow! Add *Agni Sara* as you hold, anyone?

WARRIOR POSE (*Virabhadrasana*)

THE POWER OF THE POSE: Strengthens legs and pelvis muscles; improves balance and posture; brings mobility to shoulders and opens chest; provides stability and grounding.

Stand with legs wide apart. Rotate your left leg outward 90 degrees and your right leg inward 45 degrees. Turn your pelvis so that it faces diagonally to the left. Inhale, elongate through your spine as you raise your arms overhead, palms facing one another, or clasp your hands. Exhale, bend your left knee, and point it directly over your toes (don't collapse the arch and roll inward). Sense both the upward and downward energy you need to maintain a strong, fully expanded pose. Breathe fully and hold for a minimum of three breaths. To come out of the pose, inhale to extend your left leg and turn it forward. Exhale to step your feet together, lowering your arms. Repeat facing right, bending your right knee.

MAKE IT EASIER: Supported Warrior Pose (see pregnancy section in chapter 8). If you're pregnant or unable to hold the pose standing but still want the benefit, use a sturdy chair. Sit sideways on a chair with your left side to the

your yoga coach says . . .

When you perform the Warrior Pose, be sure to keep your front knee aligned over your foot. A common error is to drop the arch and roll inward. This tendency is particularly common in women, because for most women, the line of force from the hip to the knee angles inward. To remedy this tendency, feel the sole of your natural footprint against the floor evenly. Allow the energy of the pose to travel through both your inner (tibia) and outer (fibula) leg bones.

chair's back. Extend your right leg behind, opening that hip. Extend your arms to the sides at shoulder height and look over your left hand.

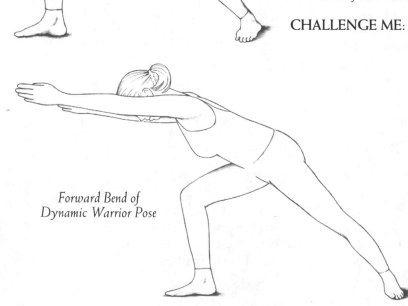

Warrior Pose

Forward Bend of Dynamic Warrior Pose

I consider the moving, *vinyasa krama*, version of this pose to be more challenging than holding the posture. It's a bit like doing a leg press on a weight machine. There are two versions of this posture sequence.

VERSION 1: Dynamic Warrior Pose 1 (*Virabhadrasana Vinyasa Krama* 1). Prepare as above. Stand with your legs wide apart. Rotate your left leg outward 90 degrees and your right leg inward 45 degrees. Rotate your torso so that it faces left. Inhale, stretch upward as you raise your arms overhead, with the palms facing one another. Exhale, bend your left knee. As you bend your knee, hinge forward from your hips so that your spine and arms are parallel to the floor. Inhale, come up to the vertical position by pressing your left foot into the floor, extending your bent left leg. Repeat two more times, bending forward as you exhale and bend your knee, coming to vertical as you inhale and extend your knee.

CHALLENGE ME: Dynamic Warrior Pose 2 (*Virabhadrasana Vinyasa Krama* 2). Begin with your front knee already bent. It will remain bent throughout the practice. Inhale, raise your arms overhead. Exhale, bend forward to the parallel position. Keeping your knee bent, inhale and come up. Exhale go over, inhale come up, several times. Repeat on the other side. If you've got anything left, hold the pose!

Caution: Do not do the Abdominal Twist Pose if you have lower back or disc injury, or during pregnancy.

ABDOMINAL TWIST POSE (*Jathara Parivartanasana*)

THE POWER OF THE POSE: Strengthens all the muscles of the waist; tones liver, gall bladder, spleen, and pancreas. Stretches back and hips; tones lumbar nerves.

This is another mega-strengthening posture, so try the less challenging practice first!

VERSION 1: Lie supine with your arms perpendicular to your body on the floor, palms down. Bend your knees and bring the soles of your feet to the floor. Exhale; draw your knees up to your chest to bring your feet off the floor. Inhale; allow your knees to reach to your left side without touching the floor. Exhale; draw your knees up toward the ceiling, rolling onto the back of your pelvis. Inhale; allow your knees to twist to the right side without touching the floor. Exhale; draw your knees up toward the ceiling, bringing your entire pelvis onto the floor. Alternate several times.

Please note that this practice can be done with your breath flowing in an opposite pattern. That is, inhale when your knees come up, exhale as they lower down. I feel you gain more integrative strength in your pelvis and hips when you breathe as first described in this practice.

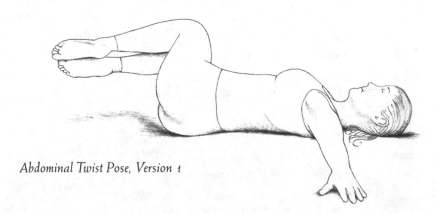

Abdominal Twist Pose, Version 1

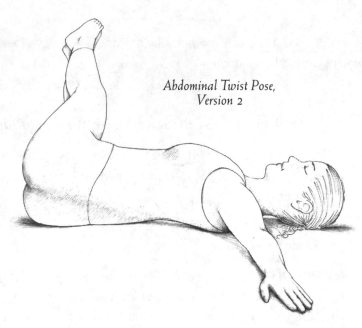

Abdominal Twist Pose,
Version 2

VERSION 2: Lie supine on your back with your arms perpendicular to your body on the floor, palms down. Exhale and bring your extended legs straight up. Inhale and rotate your extended legs left near the floor. Exhale to bring your extended legs back up toward the ceiling, rolling onto the back of your pelvis. Inhale; rotate your legs to the right side. Exhale; bring your legs back up toward the ceiling, rolling onto the back of your pelvis. Alternate several times.

CHALLENGE ME: Double Leg Lift with Solar Energizer (*Utthita Dvipadasana* with *Agni Sara*)

In this practice, you are going to put together what you have learned from other postures in this chapter. Lie on your back, arms at your sides, palms down. Perform *Agni Sara*. Exhale, draw the pelvic floor up. Squeeze your vaginal barrel and your abdominal wall sequentially from bottom to top. Inhale; release the upper, middle, and lower portions of your abdominal wall; release through your vaginal barrel and pelvic floor.

Caution: Do not do the Double Leg Lift with Solar Energizer if you have lower back or disc injury, and not during pregnancy.

balanced use of abdominal muscles

A host of muscles works synergistically throughout the pelvic center. Because of our erect human stance, the muscles in the abdominal wall require cultivation. Their strength and flexibility must be balanced with that of the muscles deep in the pelvis.

The transverse abdominal muscles are the deepest of the girdle-like muscles in the abdominal wall. Except for a central section of connective tissue, these muscles run around your abdomen horizontally, like a stack of tires. (Visualize the Michelin tire man.) To isolate the action of these muscles, relax on your spine with your knees bent, the soles of your feet on the floor. Imagine that your abdominal region is the front of a lace-up shoe. As you exhale, tighten the laces of the shoe by visualizing, and at the same time feeling, the front two sides of your pelvis narrow toward your midline. Use only as much muscular power as you need to enact this image as you breathe. Most likely you have now isolated your transverse abdominal muscles.

The internal oblique and external oblique muscles lie external to the transverse abdominal muscles and, save for a central sheath, they run diagonally upward to the midline and diagonally downward from the midline, respectively. To feel them work together, remain supine and imagine there is a cantaloupe inside your abdomen. As you exhale, gently squeeze this melon. Again, use only as much force as you need to squeeze this imaginary object. Feel the movement traveling inward toward your lower back. Now you are using your internal and external oblique muscles.

Embedded in the central connective tissue of the internal oblique muscles, the pair of *rectus abdominis* muscles is attached by tendons to the pubic bone and runs up the very center of your abdomen to the bottom of your breastbone, attaching there to sets of ribs on both sides. To feel them engage, put your chin to your chest and lift your head and upper torso off the floor. Curl the bottom of your spine, and lift up toward your navel as well. Here you are mainly using the *rectus abdominis* muscles (see illustration on page 43).

The *iliopsoas* group of muscles is made up of the *psoas major,* the *psoas minor,* and the *iliacus.* These muscles, which travel deep into the pelvis, are attached to the lower back and connect to your inner thigh. They lift your thigh bones up in front of you, or help you bend forward from the hips; and they may be very strong, even if the muscles in the front of your abdomen are not. This muscle group is primarily responsible for lifting the legs and bringing your torso to meet your thighs. In doing so, they exert some pull on your lower back. Therefore, it's important that whenever you lift your legs and whenever you sit up, you simultaneously engage the muscles of the abdominal wall. This will prevent strain in your back while strength-training your entire abdominal wall. This in turn increases stability and control, giving you more power in challenging postures and movements.

Now exhale, lift your extended legs off the floor to a 45-degree angle. Inhale and lower your legs back toward the floor, but allow them to hover an inch off the floor.

Now put the two actions together. Perform *Agni Sara* as you lift your legs while you exhale and draw up and in. Lower your legs as you inhale and release. This is not a simple practice to master. Allow yourself time to develop the subtle awareness necessary to perform this pose with dynamic internal support.

Category 2. Whole Body Integration Poses

Ever wondered how some athletes make it look easy? Or why some dancers float across the floor while others struggle? One thing the Williams sisters of the tennis world have going for them is whole body integration. As either one moves, her whole body is orchestrated to perform as efficiently as possible with a minimum of misguided action and energy. The postures below give you a chance to practice connecting each body part to and through the center. This organizational pattern underlies all the more complex movement patterns of your nervous system. When you practice these postures, visualize the area around your navel as the Grand Central Station of all the limbs, the tailbone, and the head. Explore running energy, lines of force, and information to, from, and through your navel area in each pose.

DOWNWARD-FACING BOAT POSE (*Adho Mukha Navasana*)

THE POWER OF THE POSE: Strengthens the entire back of your body, massages internal organs, and benefits abdominal glands.

Lie prone with your arms extended overhead. Inhale; simultaneously lift your arms, upper torso, and legs off the floor. As you lift into the posture, radiate energy from the navel region out in all directions. Feel a line of connection from your navel to your head, each hand, each foot, and even to your tailbone. Exhale to lower. Repeat two more times. There is considerable pressure on your navel center in this pose. If you are up to it, after inhaling, lift into the

Caution: Do not do the Downward-Facing Boat Pose during pregnancy.

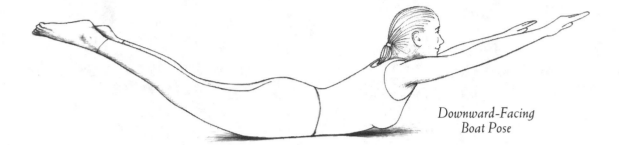

*Downward-Facing
Boat Pose*

pose. Hold while breathing evenly. Feel the energy of the pose respond to the breath rhythm. Exhale to lower whenever you're ready.

MAKE IT EASIER: If this posture is hard for you, but you still want to work to your capacity (bravo!), fold a firm blanket and place it under your pelvis and stomach region. Rest over this support first to lengthen your back muscles, and ever so gently *lengthen* your spine head-ward and tail-ward simultaneously as you lift your legs and arms. This ought to bring you to a flat position. Don't go any higher. Exhale to lower from here when ready. This may be enough. As you practice over time and this feels easier, go to the variations below without the blanket support.

Four other ways to gently approach this pose are:

1. Lift only your legs off the floor.

2. Lift only your upper body and arms.

3. Lift along the right side of your body, right arm, and leg.

4. Lift along the left side of your body, left arm, and leg.

EXTENDED TRIANGLE POSE *(Utthita Trikonasana)*

THE POWER OF THE POSE: Strengthens the pelvic area, toning the reproductive system. Stretches the muscles of the spine, side of trunk, waist, and back of legs; increases hip joint flexibility. Strengthens legs, stimulates nervous system, and improves digestive functions.

Stand with your legs wide apart. Rotate your left leg outward 90 degrees and your right leg inward 45 degrees. Inhale; stretch your arms out to the sides at

Extended Triangle Pose

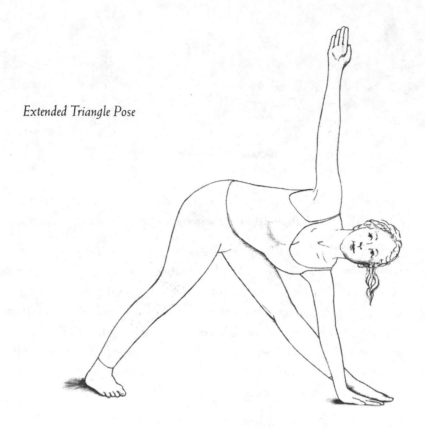

shoulder height. Feel the energy radiate out through all your limbs, head, and tailbone from your navel region. Exhale; bend flat to the left. Place your left hand on the outside of your thigh, knee, shin, or on the floor while extending your right arm upward. Breathe evenly for three or more breaths to your comfortable capacity. Inhale to come up. Exhale your arms to the sides.

MAKE IT EASIER: When your hips or hamstrings are tight, you may wish to practice the triangle pose by slightly bending the knee you bend toward. Begin with your legs wide apart. Rotate your left leg outward 90 degrees and your right inward 45 degrees. As you bend to the left, allow your left knee to bend as much as you need to feel comfortable in the posture. Repeat on the other side.

CHALLENGE ME: Perform the Triangle Pose with your feet pointed straight ahead rather than turned to the side. This stretch hits different muscles in your

guiding principle: take out the slack

While studying Body-Mind Centering, a very elegant system of body work, I learned a technique called "take out the slack," in which you locate each end of a specific tissue, such as a nerve or ligament, and ever so gently elongate it. This technique exemplifies what the entire body is to do in yoga practice. Some teachers ask you to connect or extend. Some invite you to radiate. Whatever you call it, allow your body to expand in all dimensions by activating the space inside with energy. Wake up every cell! You want every single one of those living entities to participate in your practice and to be available to your perception as it develops. When I take out the slack in yoga practice, I feel like I've turned on every light in every room in my body house. I imagine all my cells communicating, talking together (forgive me) on their cell phones.

hip and groin areas. You will not bend as far to the side. Remember to keep flat to the side rather than allowing the top shoulder to roll forward.

You can do either of these variations of the Triangle Pose without putting weight into your lower hand. This will create a more strenuous posture for your torso muscles. Explore different arm positions with your free upper arm. Try reaching your arm overhead or wrap it behind your back, palm facing outward. Also explore looking forward with your eyes softly focused, looking down toward your lower foot; or, for a balance challenge, turn your head to look up.

DOWNWARD-FACING DOG POSE (*Adho Mukha Shvanasana*)

THE POWER OF THE POSE: Stretches muscles and smoothes connective tissue throughout body. Opens the shoulders and the back, especially the backs of the legs; has properties of inverted poses.

Begin on your hands and knees, placing your hands slightly forward of your shoulders. Inhale to turn your toes under. Exhale to push with your hands while you reach your tailbone up and back on a diagonal. With some luck, this action will bring you to your hands and feet with your pelvis high. With your knees slightly bent and your heels off the floor, lengthen your entire torso by stretching your arms out of your shoulder joints. Open your armpits. Reach

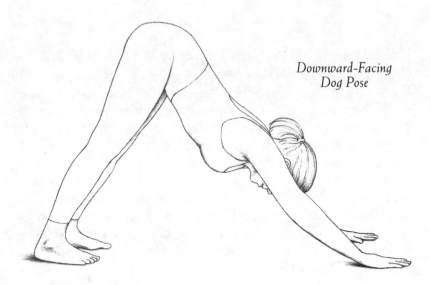

*Downward-Facing
Dog Pose*

up and back with the sitting bones. If you are able to keep your back flat or slightly arched, allow the top of your head to aim toward the floor while keeping your armpits open.

MAKE IT EASIER: If this pose is just too difficult either for the hamstrings and calves or for the upper body, try this less demanding alternative:

Begin on your hands and knees with your hands placed slightly forward of your shoulders. Inhale to turn your toes under. Slide your hands forward along the floor, one at a time, until your arms are both stretched out in front of you, elbows lifted. Draw your hips away from your hands, bringing your forehead to the floor. If your neck and shoulders are not the issue, bring your chin to the floor and allow your spine to arch. Work for a resilient stretch, not congestion in your shoulders.

FOUR-LIMB STAFF POSE (*Chaturanga Dandasana*)

THE POWER OF THE POSE: Strengthens muscles of the wrists, arms, shoulders, chest, and entire torso. Balances interaction between front and back spinal muscles and in general balances the nervous system. Tones abdominal organs.

From hands and knees, clasp your fingers, placing your forearms on the floor to make a triangular shape. Walk your knees away from your arms. See if you can lift one knee off the floor at a time, tucking your toes under to hold your

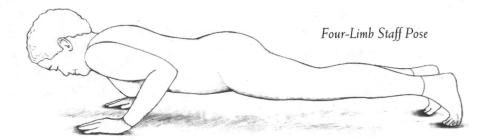

Four-Limb Staff Pose

body's weight between your elbows and your knee and toes. Try it with the other knee off the floor. Hold and breathe evenly. You get to try out the guiding principles here, because this pose takes what you've got. The idea is to keep your body stiff like a staff—hence the posture's name—so use your abdominals, radiate, connect to integrate your whole body, and keep those shoulder blades down on your back.

Next, see if you can lift both knees off the floor, holding the weight on both hands and both feet, toes tucked under. You'll eventually want your body elongated, flat, and hovering slightly above the floor. If this is really hard, lift your pelvis up a bit. As your upper body region gets stronger, you will gradually be able to lower your pelvis. (Note: this variation is not shown.)

CHALLENGE ME: This next variation requires even more integral strength throughout your entire torso. Place your palms on the floor by the sides of your chest. Tuck your toes under. Exhale to raise your whole body an inch or so off the floor. You'll be suspended on your hands and feet. If you can't yet manage to stay low, just lift your pelvis higher. You can work your way down as your core and arm strength improve. Hold initially for three breaths. This is a potent whole body strengthener that will not give you bulk, just power.

SIDE PLANK POSE (*Vasisthasana*)

THE POWER OF THE POSE: Strengthens muscles of the arms, shoulders, and spine; improves balance.

Visualize this pose before attempting it. Begin with the Downward-Facing Dog Pose. Turn your entire body in one piece to the left. Bring your right arm upward and out to the side at shoulder height. Your left leg will end up on top of your right leg. Your weight will be supported on your right hand and the outer edge of your right foot. If you want more adventure, raise your left leg up, turning it out at your hip joint. Catch hold of your large toe (or really any-thing you can out there). See if this left leg will straighten. You may want to turn your head up to look at this amazing thing you are doing. This also can help you to balance if you plan to stay here awhile. As always, three deep even breaths are good for starters. Then do the pose on the other side.

Category 3. Balance Poses

Balance postures require the full body integration practiced in the Side Plank Pose above. In fact, there is really no technical distinction, but there is instead a matter of emphasis.

THE POWER OF THE POSE: All balance poses improve your neuromus-cular system's facility in keeping you upright. The reflexive patterns that are hardwired into your nervous system are reinforced through practice. This is a "use it, don't lose it" situation. Additionally, the body areas involved primarily in keeping balance are strengthened, especially the small muscles of the feet and hands, while other areas are stretched in these postures. Balance postures improve concentration. Include at least one in your regular practice.

Before his students do standing dynamic poses (*vinyasa krama*), master yoga teacher Srivatsa Ramaswami has them stand in Mountain Pose with feet to-gether and breathe for at least six breaths. I first thought this was meant to be a centering time, a time of preparation. It was only after I seriously injured my right knee and spent the next six months hobbling on crutches that I un-derstood the importance of this first posture for balance. For the very young, the very old, and the very injured, standing erect is a balance challenge. Yet within this simplest of postures exists the opportunity to balance compression and elongation throughout the entire body. I realized this when I began to walk without crutches. I had completely stiffened up on one side while the other side had weakened. The patterns of tension in my body were no longer familiar. My injury taught me to use this posture to open shut-down areas and to balance my body around my spine from right to left and front to back.

MOUNTAIN POSE (*Tadasana*)

Stand with your feet hips-width apart, closer together or with insides of feet touching. Feel your weight evenly on your feet. Allow your knees to be soft, so energy can run up and down through your legs. Allow your tailbone to root

standing alignment

Here is another of many ways to explore standing alignment. Imagine a fountain coming up through your feet, legs, spine, and out the top of your head. Allow the external areas of your body to drape like water running down the sides of a fountain. Let your arms hang so your shoulders drape away from your ears. Soften your rib cage muscles with each exhalation and allow the weight of your body to drape around your fountain-like core. Release any tension you don't need to help you stand. Keep this in mind as you perform other postures.

into the ground as if it were a long lion's tail. Feel the gentle forward curve of your low back and the backward curve of your rib cage. Feel your smaller neck bones curving forward. Can you feel the place where the spine becomes the head? Gently allow your head to float up from the top of the spine. Locate areas of compression around your spine—in the front, back, and at each side. Do you know what purpose they serve or how they got there? Ask your body. Remain in the pose for a minimum of six breaths or until you're ready to transition to something else.

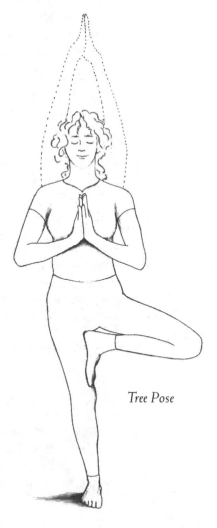

Tree Pose

TREE POSE (*Vrikshasana*)

Stand with your legs together. Rotate your left leg out to the side, bend your left knee, and place your foot on your right leg at your ankle, knee, or top of your thigh. (You may need to use your hands to place your foot in the last position.) Inhale, bring your hands to your chest, palms together, or raise them overhead, being sure not to arch your back. Breathe evenly and hold for a minimum for three breaths. Lower your hands and arms, release your foot, and relax, standing on both feet. Repeat using the other leg. It is helpful to softly focus your eyes on something in front of you.

MAKE IT EASIER: Is it hard to balance? Hold the back of a chair or lightly touch the wall.

CHALLENGE ME: Bring your hands overhead, palms together. Exhale and bend forward from your hips and touch the floor with the tips of your fingers. If you can't go that far over, just go as far as comfortable. Inhale to come up. Be sure to keep your arch lifted and your knee soft (or even slightly bent) over your toes. Do the same on the other side.

STANDING SCALE POSE (*Tolasana*)

(This posture is sometimes considered a variation of the Warrior Pose [*Virabhadrasana*]. Here we are going to approach *Tolasana* as a scale that balances the forward body weight with the backward body weight.)

     Stand with your feet close together. Inhale; raise your arms overhead, palms facing one another. Exhale; bend forward from your right hip as you bring your

guiding principle: dig in!

Imagine a walk in bare feet on moist soft grass. Now picture a walk in heeled boots on ice. In the first case, you are grounding your energy into the earth. In the second case, you are not. You are drawing your energy up and holding it in your body so as not to slip and fall on the ice. In yoga practice, you want to ground your body, as in the first example, by yielding its weight into the earth. This doesn't mean you should collapse like a rag doll. To yield means to transfer some of your weight into the ground, just like a plant sending down roots. The plant maintains its structural form above the root. The root then gives the plant more stability and support.

Try this: Stand and think of your body as sealed off by the skin all the way around. Imagine you are teetering on something very narrow and slippery. Take a short walk around. How do you feel? Uprooted? Cut off? Now stand and open your periphery, feel porous through your skin. Feel your feet spread into that soft grassy carpet, or use the image of warm sand. Take a walk. Let your feet relax and your weight sink in. Sense whatever is under the floor. Do you notice a feeling of support rising up through your bones in return? This is the feeling to go for in your practice. Root with the parts of your body that touch the floor in holding any pose. Allow the points of contact to radiate support in return into the structures of your body.

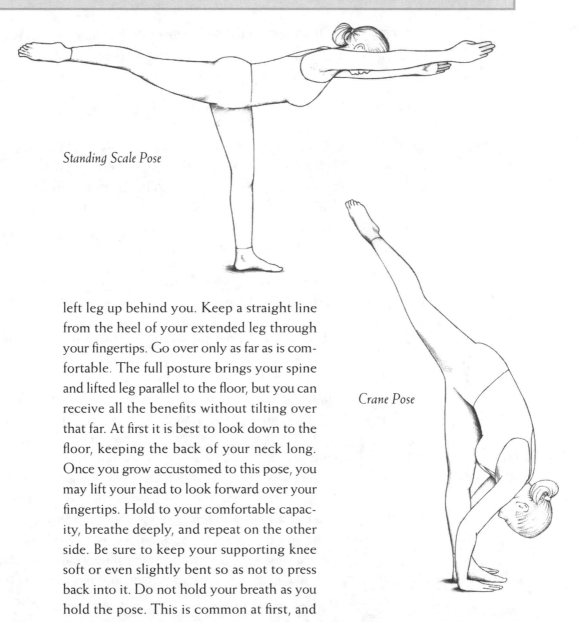

Caution: Do not do the Standing Scale Pose if you have high blood pressure.

Standing Scale Pose

Crane Pose

left leg up behind you. Keep a straight line from the heel of your extended leg through your fingertips. Go over only as far as is comfortable. The full posture brings your spine and lifted leg parallel to the floor, but you can receive all the benefits without tilting over that far. At first it is best to look down to the floor, keeping the back of your neck long. Once you grow accustomed to this pose, you may lift your head to look forward over your fingertips. Hold to your comfortable capacity, breathe deeply, and repeat on the other side. Be sure to keep your supporting knee soft or even slightly bent so as not to press back into it. Do not hold your breath as you hold the pose. This is common at first, and it indicates that you may not be focusing on feeling the supporting leg's connection to the ground. Feel your weight transfer into and out of the ground through your supporting leg. Lengthen along the lines of the posture and relax.

MAKE IT EASIER: If it's hard to balance at first, place a chair, with its back toward you, a few feet in front of you. Lightly hold the back of the chair as you bend forward for a more secure balance.

CHALLENGE ME: Crane Pose (*Bakasana*)

From the Standing Scale Pose, continue to plunge forward until your fingertips or palms rest on the floor. At the same time, gently lift your extended leg. If this is easy, then continue to lower your chest until you fold at your hips, placing your chest against your supporting leg, hands around the back of your heel. Can you lift your extended leg straight up?

EXTENDED HAND-TO-BIG-TOE POSE (*Utthita Hasta Padangusthasana*)

VERSION 1: Extended Hand-to-Big-Toe Pose (*Utthita Hasta Padangusthasana*)—Forward. The supporting leg is usually extended in this pose, but I feel it is easier to find the correct alignment if you bend it to get started. Stand on two feet. Exhale, bend your knees, and shift the weight onto your left foot. Flex at your hip to bring your right knee up. Catch hold of it, wrapping your hand around the forward portion of your knee. Inhale, stretch up through your spine, and straighten the supporting knee (only if this is comfortable). You may also wish to bring your left arm up over your head to support the sense of elongation. Sometimes it's fun to explore a hand gesture or *mudra* in this pose. Fold your index and middle fingers down to meet your thumb, leaving the

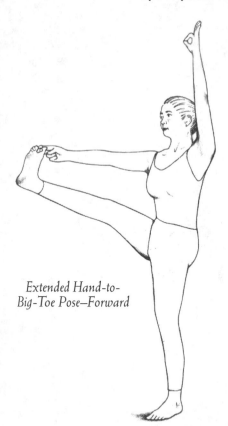

Extended Hand-to-Big-Toe Pose—Forward

fourth and fifth finger stretching upward. Breathe evenly for three breaths or more to your comfortable capacity. Exhale to bring your arms and legs back down. Repeat on the other side.

To try a different variation, instead of holding your knee, turn your lifted leg out slightly and grab hold of your big toe—hence the posture's name.

CHALLENGE ME: The final variation of the pose requires extension in both legs. Stand with both legs together. Bend your knees and shift your weight to your left foot. Bring your right knee up and grab hold of your right toe. Inhale, extend in three directions simultaneously. Press down through your left foot to extend the left supporting leg. Reach out through your right foot to extend your right leg. Reach your left arm upward to extend along your spine and torso. As you maintain the pose, check to see that you are making a good footprint, with the arch of your supporting foot lifted and your toes spread out on the floor. Keep your tailbone rooted into the ground so that your low back can stretch. If you just can't stand to hold on to that big toe, you can grab hold of your foot, wrapping your palm around the outside edge. Repeat on the other side.

VERSION 2: Extended Hand-to-Big-Toe Pose (*Utthita Hasta Padangusthasana*)—Side. This version of the posture simply brings the lifted leg out to the side. Go through the same procedure as above, but instead of straightening your leg in front of your body, follow the turnout of the hip and extend your leg to the side. Bring your free arm out to the opposite side at shoulder height. If you would like to explore a hand gesture (*mudra*) in your free hand, reach your middle finger down to the ground while extending through your other four fingers.

KING DANCER POSE (*Natarajasana*)

VERSION 1. From standing, exhale and bend both knees. Shift the weight onto your left foot. At the same time, bend your right knee and grasp your foot behind your pelvis. Inhale; lift your left arm overhead, reaching your tailbone down to the ground and keeping your right knee next to your left knee. If you feel no pressure in your right knee, you may gently pull your heel toward your buttocks. Softly focus your eyes on

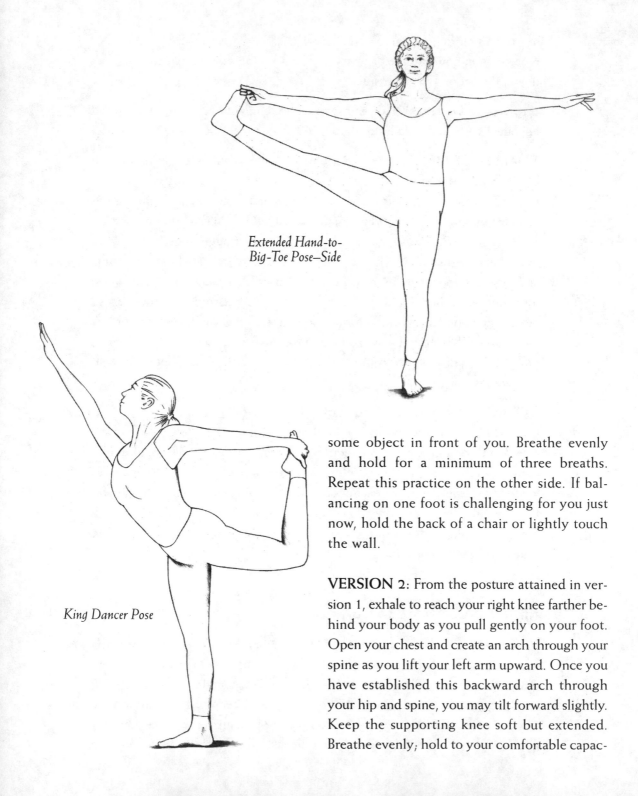

*Extended Hand-to-
Big-Toe Pose–Side*

King Dancer Pose

some object in front of you. Breathe evenly and hold for a minimum of three breaths. Repeat this practice on the other side. If balancing on one foot is challenging for you just now, hold the back of a chair or lightly touch the wall.

VERSION 2: From the posture attained in version 1, exhale to reach your right knee farther behind your body as you pull gently on your foot. Open your chest and create an arch through your spine as you lift your left arm upward. Once you have established this backward arch through your hip and spine, you may tilt forward slightly. Keep the supporting knee soft but extended. Breathe evenly; hold to your comfortable capac-

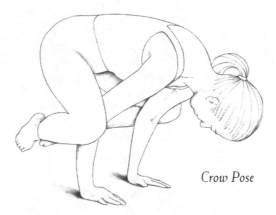

Crow Pose

ity. Return to the version 1 position on an inhalation. Exhale and lower your leg and arms. Repeat on the other side.

CROW POSE (*Bhujapidasana*)

Here's a balance pose that improves upper body strength. Stand with your legs hips-width apart. Squat down and place your palms on the floor in front of you. Place your upper thighs on your upper arms. This feels like you're tucking your elbow into the crease behind your knee. Shift your weight forward over your palms and slowly lift your toes off the floor. (Don't hold your breath.) Hold the pose for five to ten seconds. Shift back to return your feet to the floor. You may wish to shake your hands or circle your wrists after finishing the posture.

MAKE IT EASIER: The Crow Pose requires a great deal of integrated strength in the muscles of the back and shoulders, not to mention the arms, hands, and wrists. Also, as in any balance pose, there is a fear factor. You may not want to topple onto your nose. Some students place a small pillow or folded blanket on the floor in front of them. You can also practice this pose without lifting your toes off the floor.

Squat down and place your hands in front of your face. Bend your elbows so you get your face closer to the floor. Come up onto the balls of your feet and tilt forward so you feel weight in both of your hands. Tilt far enough forward so you can press down into the ground with your hands. Breathe as fully as possible and stay to your comfortable capacity. Then just push back so your weight returns to your feet in a squatting position. You may wish to repeat this several times. If you practice it regularly, you will surprise yourself one day and push right into the pose without thinking about it!

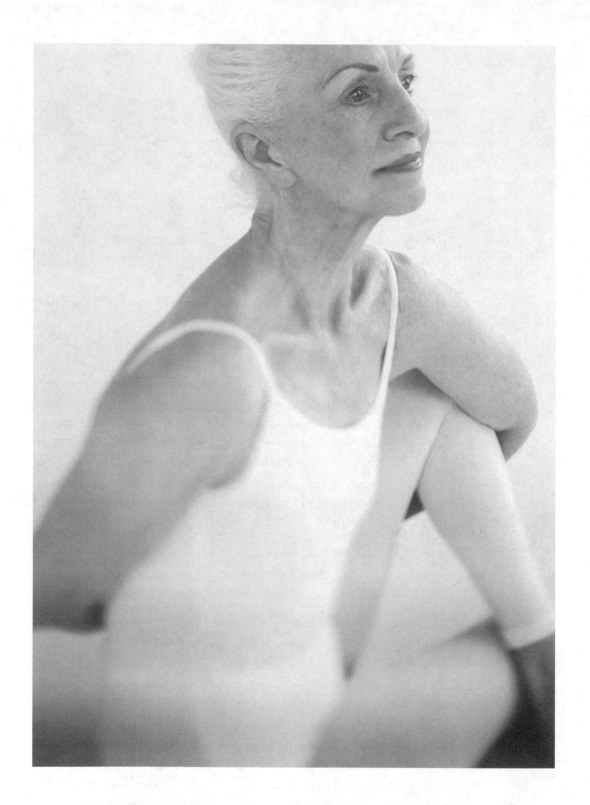

chapter 4

the essential postures for women II
bending, mobility, and twisting poses

Asana *practice will help a person endure and even minimize the external influences on the body such as age, climate, diet, and work.*
—Yoga Sutras of Patanjali, 2.48

In a single hatha *session you pass through the entire cycle of reincarnation, . . . having been a tree, a locust, a child, a warrior, a corpse, and the entire cycle of creation, preservation, and destruction.*
—Swami Veda

Category 4. Side-Bending Poses

Side-bending poses directly benefit the organs in the torso, and for this reason they are important. You may run, lift weights, power walk, or cycle, but in all of these fitness modalities, you never once bend sideways. Side bends alleviate tension in the deep muscles of the back and waist and help open your hips. I have seen a knee problem in a cyclist who overused his lateral muscles from his waist to his ankles disappear through a steady therapeutic side-bending yoga program. If you are like most people, you use your dominant hand side for almost everything you do. Side bends help to balance many patterns and are especially good for string musicians, tennis players, carpenters, and other victims of one-handed repetitive strain.

ABDOMINAL STRETCH POSE (*Jathara Parivritta*)

Lie supine with legs together, arms out to the sides at shoulder height, palms down. Move your legs incrementally to the right along the floor. This will create a long curve through your body. Stop when you feel an intense stretch along the left side of your torso and hip. Turn your head to the left. Relax the feet and shins once you have established the posture. Breathe and relax. To come out of the pose, turn your face upward and incrementally walk your heels back to the starting position. Repeat by walking your heels over to the left side and turning your face to the right. This is a deceptively intense stretch, so be mindful of how far to the side you place your legs.

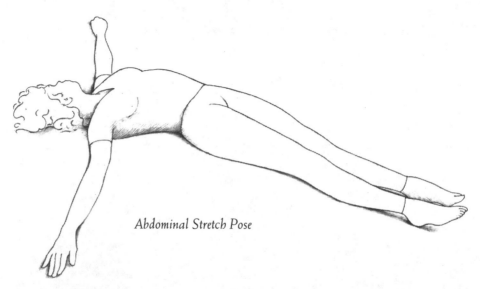

Abdominal Stretch Pose

SERPENT SIDE-BEND SERIES (*Anantasana*)

(This one is particularly good for relieving neck tension.)

Lie on your left side with your left arm stretched over your head along the floor. Bend your knees slightly and place your right hand on the floor for balance. This is a series of four side bends that alternates the stretch from one side to the other.

1. Bring your left arm out in front of you at shoulder height along the floor. Allow the side of your head to touch the floor so that the right side of your neck stretches. You may want to wrap your right arm around your back, bending your right elbow, palm facing outward. For balance, you could place these fingertips on the floor. Hold and breathe.

2. We're going to bend your spine in the opposite direction. Bring your left elbow to the floor and place the left side of your head above your ear in the palm of your left hand. Relax your neck and shoulders and let your spine drape between your hand and your lower ribs. Hold and breathe.

3. Lift your torso up and bring your left elbow underneath your ribs or left shoulder. Allow your head to aim toward the floor. Inhale to lift

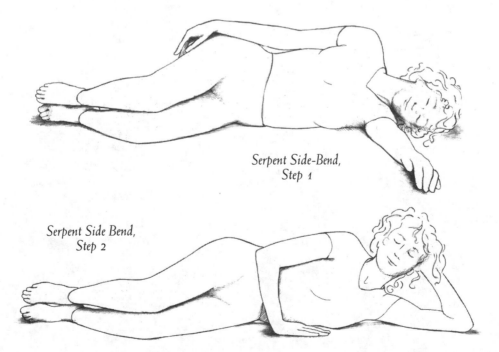

Serpent Side-Bend,
Step 1

Serpent Side Bend,
Step 2

your right arm up to the ceiling, then over your head, keeping the upper arm near your right ear as you bend to the left. Lift upward through your lower ribs. Feel a long arc, like a low mound or bridge from your right hip to the fingertips of your right hand.

4. Finally, lift your head upward, reversing the curve once more. Bring the palm of your left hand to the floor near your left hip and push down gently through that arm to extend upward. You may bend your right knee or both knees so as to allow your waist to drape toward the floor from your left hip to your left shoulder.

Repeat the sequence on the other side.

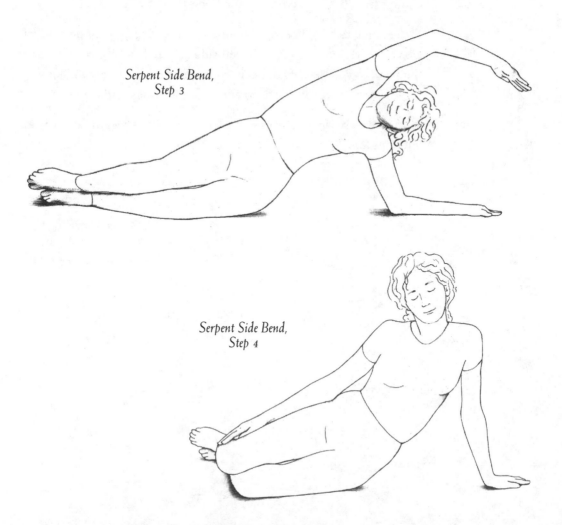

Serpent Side Bend,
Step 3

Serpent Side Bend,
Step 4

guiding principle: breathe into it

You're in the pose, focusing on the breath. Now what? Imagine the life energy, or *prana,* swirling into the stretched areas. See it as sunlight, or hear a sound such as "Om." Or imagine that part of the body breathing. And, of course, it is breathing! Every cell in your body is constantly taking in nutrients and expelling waste, organs are filling and emptying, fluids are transporting substances here and there. When you imagine breath flowing through a stretched area, or imagine that body part (say, your foot) breathing, you support the body's ability to nurture, open, and cleanse that place with vital force.

SITTING SIDE BEND (*Parshvottanasana*) WITH NECK WORK

This posture is a good preparation for all side-bending poses while being an intense side stretch itself. Sit with your legs crossed. You can also do this practice sitting in a chair. Inhale; raise your arms overhead, palms facing one another. Exhale, clasp your hands behind your head, or touch the back of your head, elbows back and out to the sides. Feel the stretch across your chest and shoulders. Inhale; lift your left elbow up as you bend to the right, stretching the left side of your body. Press the sitting bones into the floor and lift your ribs. You may bring your right hand down to the floor or chair seat, but keep

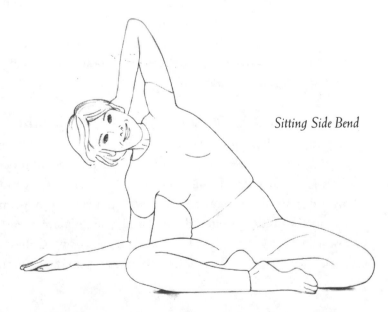

Sitting Side Bend

your yoga coach says . . .

The most common error in side bending is to allow your torso to roll forward so that you aren't flat to the side. Not surprisingly, the Sanskrit word for some side bends translates to "twist." This is a helpful suggestion. As you bend to the side, twist the side you are bending toward slightly forward, and the side that will receive the stretch slightly backward. A helpful trick: Rotate the palm of the side you are bending toward upward. Reach from your little finger and let it stretch the bottom tip of your shoulder blade out away from your spine. Now bend to the side, keeping this rotation. Do you feel flatter to your side?

this elbow bent. If your torso permits, bring your right elbow down to the floor. Keep both sitting bones on the floor. Try changing the position of your upper left arm by wrapping it behind your back, palm facing outward. Do a long reach from your head to come up as you inhale. If you have been in the pose for a long time, come out by rolling forward so that your chest faces downward over your folded legs. Next, roll up, feeling the support of your bones in your pelvis and spine. Repeat on the other side.

Focus on your neck. Bend to the right side as above, but instead of reaching your left elbow upward, extend your left arm down along the left side of your body. Reach your shoulder away from your ear. Let your head hang away from the arm to the right. You may decide to turn your nose slowly toward your right shoulder. Adding small movements, like rolling your shoulder or your head or both, can help to gently encourage muscles in your neck and upper torso region to loosen up.

HEAD-TO-KNEE POSE (*Janu Shirshasana*)—SIDE

Sit with your legs spread wide. Bend your left knee and bring your heel close to your pelvis. Inhale and raise both arms to the sides at shoulder height. Twist slightly to the left to bring your right shoulder blade forward. Exhale; bend toward your right extended leg. Place your right arm, palm up, on the floor against the inside of your right leg. Bring your left arm over your head to reach toward your right foot. Feel flat and open across your chest. Do not roll your upper left shoulder forward. Lengthen through your neck, feel the weight of

neck rolls

Although we talk about the neck as if it were an isolated body part, in practice it is best to recognize it as the upper part of the spine. Neck rolls are often given as the main way to work with the neck. This can be fine for some and hazardous for others, depending on a number of factors, such as the state of tension in the neck muscles and the way the individual is accustomed to holding and moving her head. Neck mobility involves the entire spine. Work with your neck by sensing the entire spine and the movement possibilities throughout your entire torso. When you move from the neck area, always lengthen your upper spine so you decompress it as you move. Freedom of movement in your neck requires opening and mobility throughout your chest and shoulders.

the head, and allow the muscles and organs at your waist to soften. As you breathe and relax in the pose, you may find you can reach a bit farther. If possible, bring the fingertips of both hands around the sole of your foot (your right fingers reach under your heel, your left fingers reach around your toes). To come up, lengthen through your spine and push down through your hip as you inhale. When your spine returns to the vertical position, exhale and lower your arms. Arrange your legs for the posture on the other side.

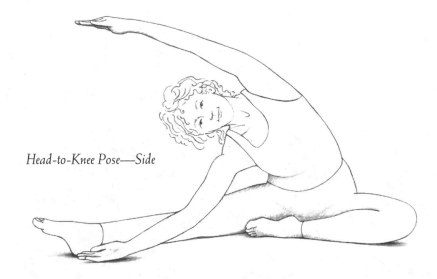

Head-to-Knee Pose—Side

HALF MOON POSE (*Ardha Chandrasana*)

Stand with your feet hips-width apart. Inhale; raise your right arm overhead. Exhale; reach up and over to the left as you bend to your left side. Try to remain flat, not allowing your body to round forward. Keep your elbow as straight as you can. Breathe evenly for three or more breaths. Inhale to return to an upright position. Exhale; lower your arm. Repeat on the other side. To intensify this posture, lift both arms.

EXTENDED SIDE-ANGLE POSE (*Utthita Parshvakonasana*)

Stand with your legs wide, toes facing forward, arms extended out to the sides. Turn your left foot out 90 degrees and your right foot in 45 degrees. Your heel will be in line with your right instep. Inhale; extend outward through your entire body. Exhale; bend your right knee, keeping your shin perpendicular to the floor. Inhale; lift your left arm up over your head as you bend to the right. Exhale; lower your right palm to the floor in front of the right instep. If you already know this is not going to be possible, just bring your right elbow onto your bent knee. Breathe evenly for three breaths or more. When you're ready to come out of the pose, inhale and come up as you push through the right foot to extend your leg. Be clear about changing the direction of your feet when you repeat the pose on the opposite side.

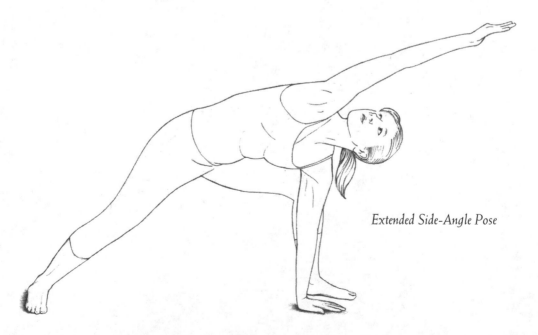

Extended Side-Angle Pose

Category 5. Shoulder Mobility and Backward-Bending Poses

Envision the standard posture of the Western world—slumped forward, shoulders rounded inward. My daughter in third grade is already showing these signs of long hours of tedium at her school desk. These postures are grouped together because they offer opening into the space around your body.

Shoulder Mobility

TWIST TO FLAPPING FISH POSTURE LOOP (*Matsya Kridasana* to *Shava Udarakarshanasana Vinyasa Krama*)

This dynamic practice (*vinyasa krama*) links two postures with breath and movement. Lying prone, bend your right arm and right leg. Turn your face to the right into the next posture, the Flapping Fish Pose.

Inhale, reach your right arm overhead, and let your arm continue to circle behind you, leading your torso into a twist. Allow your arm to continue to trace a circle down over your hips and finally forward and back to its starting position. As your arm draws a huge circle, twist at your waist so your rib cage turns from the side to the back and to the side again. Keep your fingertips close to, if not brushing, the floor. Your right knee remains bent in its starting position. Circle your arm in this direction three or more times. Rest briefly, then reverse the direction of your arm circles. Allow your shoulder to rotate freely. The more relaxed you can allow your body to be in this pose, the more benefit you will gain. To switch sides, roll onto your belly into the full Crocodile Pose. Then bend your left knee and left elbow, and turn your head to

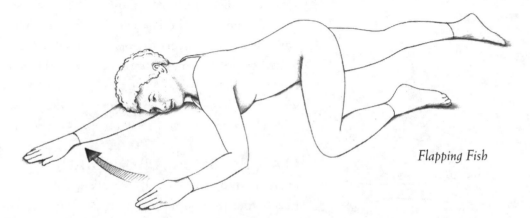

Flapping Fish

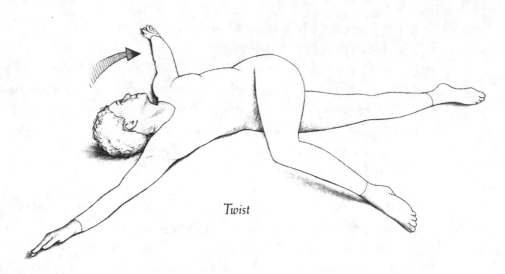

Twist

that side to rest in the Flapping Fish Pose before continuing the motion with the left arm.

The next three stretches can be done standing or sitting on the floor. Stand if it is difficult to sit on the floor while keeping your spine erect. These arm variations can be applied to a variety of poses, such as forward bends.

ELBOWS CROSS IN FRONT

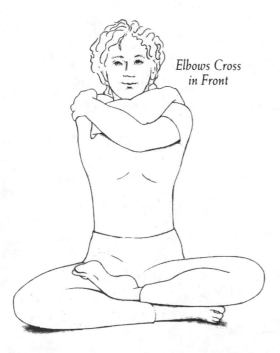

Elbows Cross in Front

Inhale, open your chest, and reach your arms backward like a bird in flight. Exhale and cross your arms in front, reaching to your opposite shoulder, elbows one on top of the other. Inhale, reach your arms open, and open your chest. Exhale, cross your other arm on top, and touch the opposite shoulder. Repeat several times. On the last exhalation, cross your arms, reach your fingers to opposite shoulders, and hold the pose. You may intensify the stretch by lifting your elbows as you inhale and lowering them as you exhale. Also draw a large circle with the elbows as you breathe in and out. Switch elbows to repeat.

CLASP HANDS: ONE UP, ONE DOWN

Have a strap, dish towel, or sock within reach. Reach your right arm up and your left arm down.

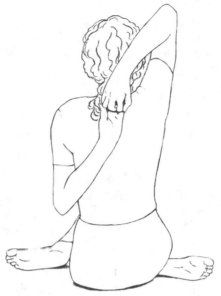

Clasp Hands:
One Up, One Down

Clasp Hands:
Low Behind Back

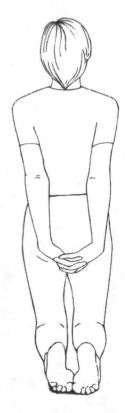

Bend both elbows to clasp your fingers behind your back. If your hands don't reach, use a strap, dish towel, or sock. Elongate through your spine. Resist the temptation to let your right elbow collapse forward. After several breaths, release. Roll your shoulders a few times and then repeat with the opposite arm position.

CLASP HANDS: LOW BEHIND BACK

Clasp your hands behind your back, interweaving your fingers. Pull your shoulder blades down and together, creating a hollow ridge between them. Use a strap if your hands do not yet comfortably clasp around your back. Lift your chin, and then lengthen through your spine. Intensify the stretch by lifting your hands away from your pelvis while bending forward.

TABLE TOP POSE (*Catuspada Pitham*)

THE POWER OF THE POSE: Along with providing mobility to the shoulders, these next two poses strengthen the arms and legs and stretch all the muscles along the front of the body. They also improve balance and concentration.

MAKE IT EASIER AND INTRODUCTION TO FULL POSE: Begin by sitting with your legs extended out in front. Place your palms on the floor behind you, fingertips pointing toward your pelvis. Lean back. Bend your knees and put the soles of your feet on the floor. If you already feel an intense stretch, you're not alone! Stop here. This is the pose. For a bit more, inhale and arch your spine, open your chest, and reach your face upward toward the ceiling. Stay within your comfortable capacity, breathing evenly. Exhale and lower your chest, looking forward. Inhale and sit up on your pelvis, extending your legs.

For the full pose, begin by sitting with your legs extended out in front. Lean back, palms on the floor behind you, fingertips pointing toward your pelvis. Bend your knees and bring the soles of your feet on the floor. Inhale, scoop your tailbone under and up while pushing down on both hands and both feet. Lengthen your head out of your spine. Do not drop it back as you hold the pose. Breathe evenly. To finish, exhale and bring your pelvis back on the floor. Inhale and sit up on your pelvis, extending your legs.

UPWARD-FACING PLANK POSE (*Purvottanasana*)

Sit with your legs extended in front. Place your palms on the floor behind you, fingertips pointing toward your pelvis. Inhale to press your palms into the floor, sliding your shoulder blades downward. Exhale to scoop your tailbone under and up while pushing down on both hands and feet; but this time, keep your legs straight. You may tilt your head back, but don't completely release

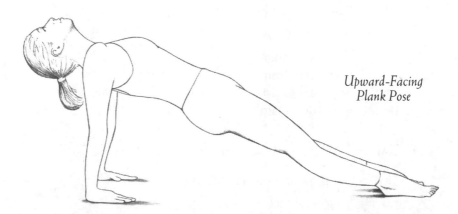

*Upward-Facing
Plank Pose*

it backward. Breathe and hold. Lower on an exhalation to the seated pose (*Dandasana*). Repeat if you like. You may also try pointing your fingers out to the sides for a slightly different stretch.

Backward Bending

Everyone should use caution regarding backward bending. For example, it does not give much benefit during pregnancy when weighed against the damage it can do. What one is capable of at this time depends on the individual. It is best to be conservative and locate a yoga teacher who has experience with yoga for pregnancy to get specific directions. Of the backward-bending postures described here, only the Half Fish Pose is generally recommended.

COBRA POSE (*Bhujangasana*)

THE POWER OF THE POSE: Strengthens back muscles and makes spine supple, stretches entire front of body, massages all torso organs, tones spinal nerves, regulates adrenals, opens chest (improving depth of breath), and improves digestion.

Caution: Do not do the Cobra Pose if you have a stomach or duodenal ulcer, a hernia, or hyperthyroidism.

guiding principle: think evolution!

All the yoga postures already exist in your body. Even if you are disabled or have passed the age where certain postures are possible, their potential is hardwired into your physiological makeup.

One myth that illustrates this feature of yoga depicts Lord Shiva observing all the animals in the world. From this study, he devised the yoga poses, which are said to number 8,400,000, with 84 central ones. When you practice a posture, you're calling it up from a large well of collective experience you share with all creatures on earth. Each posture gives a specific experience of what it is like to have your body organized in a precise way. Approach your practice as if you are calling up these parts of your larger self. I promise you will tap into something that transcends the confines of your yoga mat.

When I teach this pose, I tell students they will see current yoga books with people demonstrating this posture in a most injurious way. The models will have their shoulders up to their ears, which compresses the neck and upper torso area. (If one has chronic muscle tension there, as most mere mortals do, the nerves running through these tissues can be pinched. Ouch!). At the same time, the models will have fully extended arms and a droopy unsupported spine. This puts enormous pressure on the discs of the lower back (double-ouch! and potentially damaging). You may see advanced practitioners of yoga do the pose with this much arch. However, if they're doing it properly, they have an extended supported spine arched evenly throughout the torso. Please begin with the first variation and proceed carefully into the other more advanced ones.

Lie on the floor facing downward with your palms on the floor, fingertips in line with your nipples, and your forehead touching the floor. Exhale, reach your mouth (yes, your mouth) forward so that you feel a stretch in your throat. Inhale, peel your body off the floor, one vertebra at a time, leading with the top of your head. Allow the muscles of your back and torso to engage and lift you off the floor. In this version, do not press on your palms to go higher. Stay relatively close to the floor. Hold to your comfortable capacity and slowly lower your upper torso as you exhale. This will strengthen your upper back and neck muscles, improving your posture. If holding the pose is difficult, then simply inhale while rolling up and exhale while rolling down several times. When you finish the posture, turn your head to the side and bring your arms to the sides to rest.

MAKE IT EASIER: Bring your elbows next to your nipples with your forearms on the floor. This will decrease the amount of arch in your spine. Even

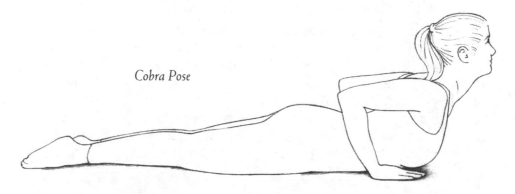

Cobra Pose

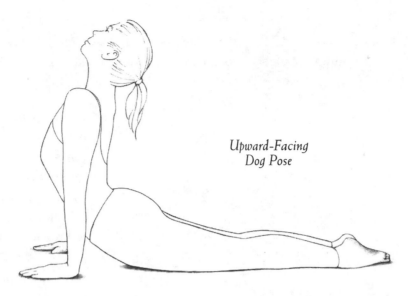

*Upward-Facing
Dog Pose*

here, press your shoulder blades down as you lift and extend through your head and neck.

CHALLENGE ME: Go through all the steps for the first variation. Now go ahead and press your palms into the floor and continue to roll back and up. Lengthen your spine. Work to feel the visceral stretch along your throat, esophagus, and stomach. Keep your elbows slightly bent unless you're able to evenly arch throughout your entire spine so your hip bones come off the floor. The fullest expression of this position is called Upward-Facing Dog Pose (*Urdhva Mukha Shvanasana*). In this pose the emphasis changes from being about reaching from the head, like a snake would, to integrating the limbs, the arms (and in some versions the legs) to support the reach of the head, like a howling dog would.

Add shoulder mobility to this backward-bending pose. Before beginning the pose, clasp your hands behind the back of your pelvis. Reach your clasped hands toward your feet to draw your shoulder blades toward one another. Slowly lift into the pose.

BOW POSE (*Dhanurasana*)

THE POWER OF THE POSE: Strengthens all back muscles; stretches abdomen; massages pancreas, reproductive organs, liver, kidneys, and adrenals.

Caution: Do not do the Bow Pose if you have high blood pressure, a stomach or duodenal ulcer, hernia, colitis, or heart weakness.

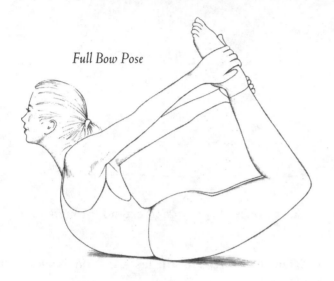

Full Bow Pose

Improves blood circulation to back and front of the body, tones spinal nerves, stimulates sympathetic nerves, and balances gland secretions. Opens the chest (increasing the depth of breath), promotes intestinal peristalsis (improving digestion), and tones reproductive organs.

The Bow Pose is an intense stretch, so let's begin with the Half Bow Pose (*Ardha Dhanurasana*). Lie prone, right arm at your side, left arm bent above your head. Bend your right knee and grasp your right ankle. Exhale to lengthen your body. Inhale and lift your head, torso, and thigh. Breathe evenly and hold. Exhale and slowly lower and release your leg. Repeat on the other side. Repeat this posture, alternating side to side three times.

For the Full Bow Pose (*Dhanurasana*), lie prone with your arms at your sides. Bend both knees and reach back to grasp your ankles one at a time. Inhale and raise your head, torso, and both thighs. You may keep your knees apart. If this is easy for you, work with them closer together. Hold. As you breathe, you may notice a slight rocking motion. Exhale and slowly lower and release your legs to the floor.

HALF PIGEON POSE (*Ardha Kapotasana*)—BACKWARD BENDING

THE POWER OF THE POSE: Rotates and stretches deep pelvic and low back muscles in an asymmetrical stretch. Opens the chest, increasing depth of breath; makes the spine supple; and opens the shoulders.

There is a huge range of variety in this pose. The main theme is the graceful arch of a bird's chest and belly recreated in the backward-bending portion of

Caution: Be careful with the Half Pigeon Pose if you have lower back problems.

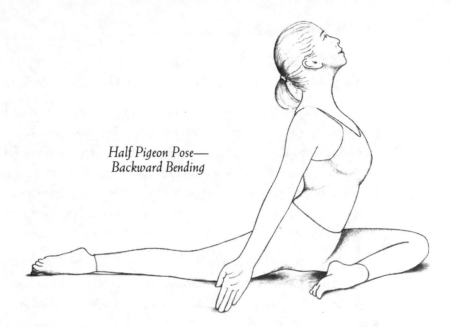

*Half Pigeon Pose—
Backward Bending*

the posture. The Full Pigeon Pose involves an extreme backward bend. Our one-sided version doesn't require such an extreme arch. However, because the pelvis is asymmetrical, the pose involves muscles in the hips, back, and torso that may not have stretched in a while (like since fifth grade), so take it easy, even if you already practice yoga.

Sit on your heels. Allow your pelvis to shift off to the left so your left heel is at your groin. Extend your right leg directly behind you, and if possible, rotate your kneecap toward the floor. Inhale; reach your arms overhead, palms together. Exhale; arch your back, bringing your chest and face up as you open your arms with your palms out to the sides. Slowly lower your fingertips to the floor behind your torso as you gently draw your shoulder blades down and together. A different arm variation is to bring your thumbs to your back on each side of your spine. Breathe fully and hold. If comfortable for your neck, lift your chin upward and then backward. Keep your neck long. Don't let your head collapse to the back. Feel your chest open. Inhale, lift from the back of your head to come up, raising your arms overhead. Repeat on the other side.

Caution: Be careful with the Monkey Pose if you have knee problems.

MONKEY POSE *(Banarasana)*

THE POWER OF THE POSE: The benefits are similar to the Half Pigeon. Slightly different muscles are used and stretched in a different arrangement.

Stand with your feet under your hips. Bend forward from your hips and shift your weight onto your left leg while slightly bending your knees. Take a long step back with your right leg, lowering into a lunge. Keep your front shin perpendicular to the floor. Depending on how your hips feel, you may choose to lift your torso up to a vertical position, placing your hands on the thigh, or raise your arms overhead to arch backward. In the later case, keep your upper arms near your ears. Breathe evenly. Repeat on the other side.

MAKE IT EASIER: If you find it hard to get into and out of this pose, use a sturdy chair for support. Stand in front of a chair, facing sideways. Bend over to place your hands on the seat as you step back to a comfortable lunge position. You can drop down to your back knee as needed to get down and up.

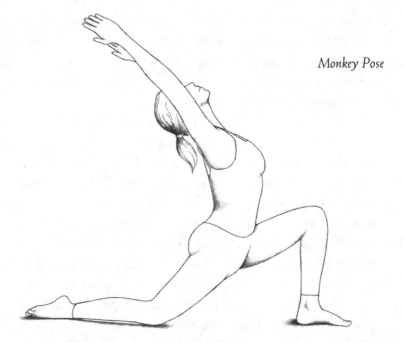

Monkey Pose

HALF FISH POSE (*Ardha Matsyasana*)

THE POWER OF THE POSE: Strengthens spine and back muscles; stretches front of neck, chest, and torso muscles and organs; stimulates thymus (boosting immune function); increases the depth of breath; and improves blood circulation in the back.

Lie supine and draw your shoulder blades together. Place your arms slightly under the back of your body with your elbows slightly bent. Push down on the back of your pelvis and your elbows to arch your spine. This will bring your head slightly off the floor; allow it to arc back. Gently relocate some weight onto the top or back of your head, depending on how arched your spine is. Breathe evenly and hold. Gently lower your body to the supine position.

MAKE IT EASIER: Roll one or two blankets into a long log. Lie back over them so they are under the bottom portions of your shoulder blades and just under your armpits.

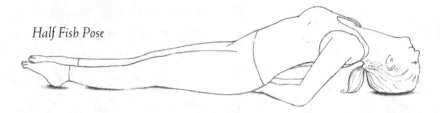

Half Fish Pose

Caution: Do not do the Half Fish Pose if you have a stomach or duodenal ulcer, hernia, heart disease, headache, or fever. Use caution if you have neck and back problems.

BRIDGE POSE (*Setu Bandhasana*)

THE POWER OF THE POSE: Strengthens spine and back muscles; stretches front of neck, chest, and torso muscles and organs; stimulates thymus-boosting immune function; increases depth of the breath; and improves blood circulation in the back.

Caution: Do not do the Bridge Pose if you have a stomach or duodenal ulcer, hernia, heart disease, headache, or fever. Use caution if you have neck and back problems.

This pose can be gotten into easily from the Desk Pose (see chapter 3, page 44). Lie supine, with knees bent, soles of the feet on the floor. Push to arch upward so just your feet, head, and upper back are on the floor. Fit your forearms, thumbs toward your spine, under your low back. If you can't lift your back high enough to fit your forearms underneath it, draw your shoulder blades together to clasp your hands behind your back on the floor, or use a strap. Another variation that may be more comfortable is to hold onto your heels.

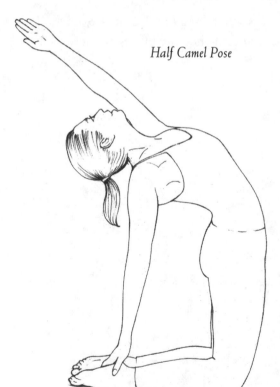

Half Camel Pose

CAMEL POSE (*Ushtrasana*)

THE POWER OF THE POSE: Intensely stretches the entire torso, muscles, organs, all tissues; opens the chest to improve breathing and correct posture; regulates thyroid.

This again is another mighty stretch. Think of the Half Camel Pose (*Ardha Ushtrasana*) as a challenging backward bend. You may never need to go any farther. Kneel with your knees slightly wider than your hips. If this is uncomfortable for your knees, fold a towel and place it under them. Turn slightly to your left and reach back to grasp your left heel with your left hand. This may be enough, in which case, wrap your right arm around your waist. Breathe and hold. Otherwise, while holding your

Caution: Do not do the Camel Pose if you have back problems.

left heel, pivot your torso so your chest faces upward, and lift your right arm overhead, with your elbow near your ear. Gently press your pelvis forward and elongate through your spine. Hold. Repeat on the other side.

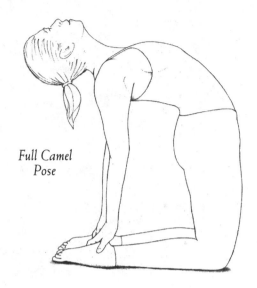

Full Camel Pose

To perform the Full Camel Pose (*Ushtrasana*), begin from the Half Camel Pose, left hand holding your left heel. Reach your right hand back to grasp your right heel. Elongate your spine as you carefully press your pubic bone forward to increase the arch. Breathe evenly. A gentle way to release the pose is to slowly sit on your heels, bringing your spine to vertical. If this posture is easy for you, repeat it with your knees kept close together.

CHALLENGE ME: Wheel Pose (*Chakrasana*)

THE POWER OF THE POSE: Gives an intense stretch to the entire front of your body, spine, and organs while strengthening the legs and arms. Improves posture, influences hormonal secretions, and improves breathing. Has properties of inverted poses.

From lying on your back, go into the Bridge Pose. Next, place your hands, palms down, with your fingertips just under your shoulders. Exhale and push your palms and feet into the floor to bring your body up into an even arch. If you're comfortable here, you may walk your hands closer to your feet. Breathe evenly. Exhale and walk your hands away and progressively lower your shoulders, back, and pelvis to the floor. You may wish to do the Child's Pose (described later in this chapter) to relax your spine in a counterposition.

Caution: Do not do the Wheel Pose if you have back problems.

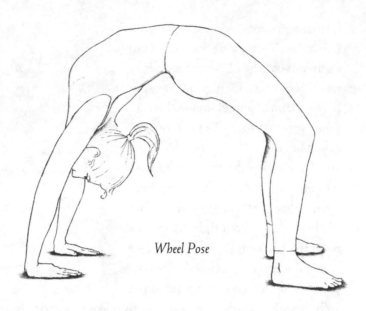

Wheel Pose

Category 6. Twisting Poses

There are several variations of twisting postures called *Matsyendrasana*. I feel that all yoga twisting postures spawn from this one. There is a wonderful story of Lord Shiva instructing his wife in yoga at the water's edge (or perhaps it was the other way around!). A fish, recognizing that these were Divine beings, kept still and quiet by the shoreline so he could listen in on what they were saying. When Shiva discovered that the fish had learned yoga, he blessed the fish and named him Matsyendra, Lord of the Fishes. The fish is said to have turned into Matsyendranath, a renowned tenth-century yogi.

But why would a royal fish be the icon for spinal twisting? An explanation exists in yoga anatomy. The currents of *prana* or life energy flow in three main channels, or *nadis*, along the spine, with thousands of tributaries. While these channels are not the physical nerves, they are similar in design, location, and function. Energy flows through the *nadis*, like fish swimming in a current, to every part of the body. This posture stimulates and helps regulate the flow of energy throughout the entire body; it is the ruler of the fish.

Western anatomy suggests that spinal twists stretch all spinal nerves be-cause they are embedded in the torso, so in this way the nervous system is ben-efited by the pose. When you stimulate all the spinal nerves, you stimulate the entire body—organs, skin, muscles, the works. Spinal twist postures are one

guiding principle: the spine in yoga practice

Some schools of yoga remind students that the point of every posture is to elongate the spine. Others visualize the spine as the main channel for the body's dynamic currents of energy. Still other approaches emphasize the spine as the axis for all coordinated movements of torso and limbs.

No matter what the emphasis is, the spine's importance in yoga practice cannot be overstated. Thirty-one pairs of spinal nerves enter and exist along its length. The loss of flexibility and strength in the muscles that move and support the spine is a major cause of injury and pain for millions of people and contributes to degeneration of the joints (discs) of the spine. Yoga practice balances the flexibility and strength of all the muscles that move the spine in every direction. Even the simplest yoga routine will elongate, twist, and bend the spine in every direction and give you a chance to relax the muscles.

Caution for All Twisting Poses: Do not do if you have a stomach or duodenal ulcer, hernia, or hyperthyroidism. Use modified practices after the second or third month of pregnancy. Use attentive care if you have sciatica or disc problems.

of the most essential categories of practice. You get a host of whole-body benefits from this single kind of posture.

THE POWER OF TWISTING POSES: In addition to toning the nerves, the muscles all along the spine and throughout the torso are stretched, and alternate abdominal organs like the kidneys are massaged. Circulation is improved, as are the hormonal secretions of affected glands, such as the adrenals. Additionally, digestion is improved.

UNIVERSAL TWIST POSE (*Shava Udarakarshanasana*)

The central idea in this twist is to keep your upper back and shoulder region on the floor while the torso twists with the legs in some arrangement. You can arrange your legs in a number of ways. Each involves slightly different muscles throughout your entire torso, hips, neck, and thighs. Where you place the

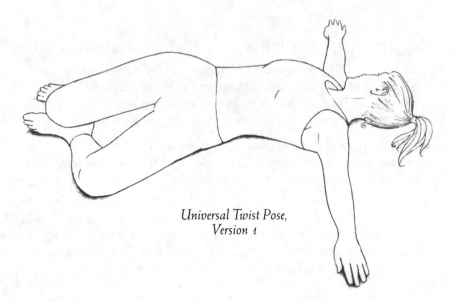

Universal Twist Pose,
Version 1

legs as they cross over to the opposite side—higher, lower, closer to, farther from the torso—creates further options for opening.

VERSION 1: Lie supine, arms out to the sides at shoulder height, knees bent, soles of your feet on the floor. Exhale, lower your knees slowly to the left as you spiral your head right. Reach outward along the floor with your right arm to keep this shoulder blade near or on the floor. When ready to release, exhale, elongate your lower spine, and bring your pelvis flat to the floor as your knees go up. Repeat on the other side.

VERSION 2: Lie supine with arms out to the sides at shoulder height, palms down. Inhale to bend your knees, lifting your feet off the floor. Exhale to lower your bent legs to the left as you spiral your face to the right. Repeat on the other side.

VERSION 3: Keeping your left leg extended on the floor, bend your right knee up to touch your toes to your left knee. Spiral through your torso as you direct your right knee to the floor across the pelvis. Keep reaching out to the right side with your right arm and spiral your face to the right.

To increase the twist, you can scoot your left hip back to reach farther across your body with your right knee. If you like, press this knee gently into the floor with your left hand. Repeat on the other side.

VERSION 4: This time extend the crossing leg and bend the underlying one.

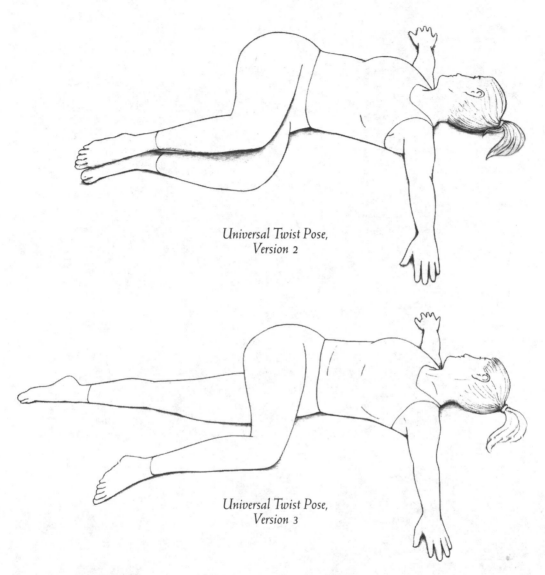

Universal Twist Pose,
Version 2

Universal Twist Pose,
Version 3

VERSION 5: This version will intensify the stretch in version 4 and add a stretch for the hamstring. Keeping your left leg extended on the floor, bend your right knee up to touch your toe to your left knee. Spiral through your spine as you direct your right knee across your pelvis. Keep reaching out to the right side with your right arm, and spiral your head to the right. Now extend your right leg. See if you can reach your hand with your toes and hold on to them.

Repeat on the other side.

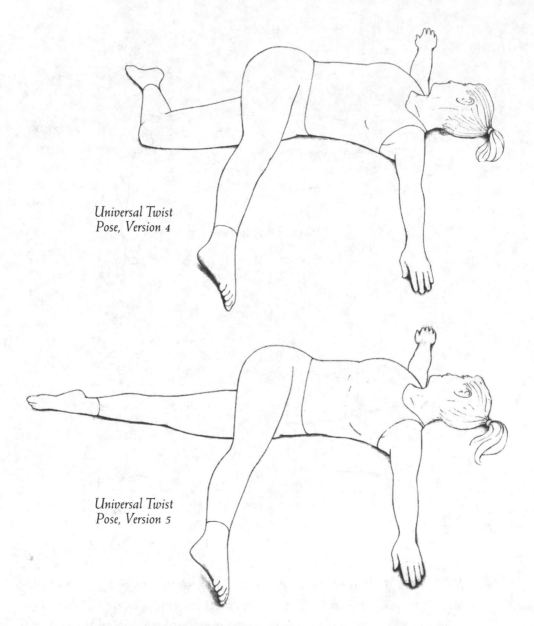

*Universal Twist
Pose, Version 4*

*Universal Twist
Pose, Version 5*

SITTING TWIST POSE (*Bharadvajasana*)

Sit with your knees bent, both feet beside your right hip. Inhale; lift your arms overhead to stretch your spine. Exhale, twist around to the left as you bring your arms down, and keep looking around to the left behind you. Sit tall and breathe deeply. To release, inhale and reach your arms overhead as you turn to the front. Exhale, bring your arms down. Repeat on the other side.

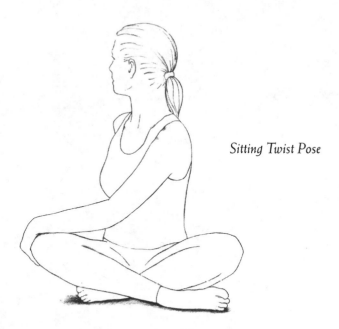

Sitting Twist Pose

MAKE IT EASIER: If you find it difficult to keep your back erect because of how your legs are arranged, just sit cross-legged. Put your other foot on top when you change sides.

CHALLENGE ME: Sit with legs extended in front. Bend your left knee and bring your left heel into the crease of your right hip, placing the foot on the

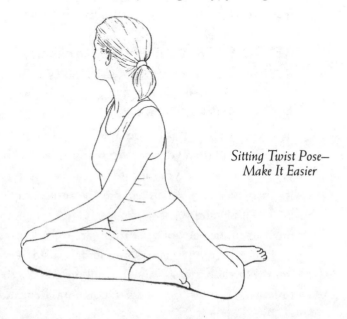

*Sitting Twist Pose—
Make It Easier*

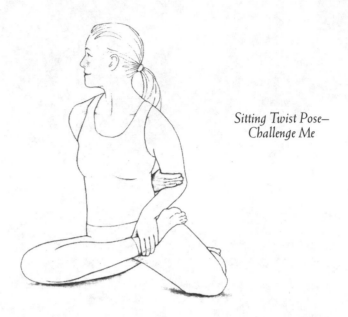

Sitting Twist Pose—
Challenge Me

topmost part of your right thigh. Rotate your right leg inward as you bend your right knee to bring this heel by your right hip. Reach your left arm behind your back around your waist to grasp your right elbow. Bring your right hand around to your left ankle. If this is easy, instead of grasping your right elbow with your left hand, reach around behind to the toes of your left foot and reach the right hand to the left knee. Turn your head to the right

REVOLVED TRIANGLE POSE (*Parivritta Trikonasana*)

Stand with legs wide, arms out to the sides, shoulder height. Turn your left leg out 90 degrees and your right leg in 45 degrees. Inhale and stretch fingertip to fingertip. Exhale and revolve this horizontal line around to the left so that now your right arm is (more or less) over your left foot. Inhale again and radiate outward from your navel center. Exhale and bend from your hips to reach your right hand to your left foot. It may not get there; in which case, place it somewhere on your left leg. Breathe and continue to radiate outward through all four limbs and *your head*. Your left knee may want to bend if your hamstring muscles in the back of your thigh are tight. Please let this happen if it needs to! Don't force your leg to straighten. Instead, relax the muscles in the back of your thigh as best you can. You will progress in the pose over time. Hold and breathe. Reverse the process to come up. Repeat on the other side.

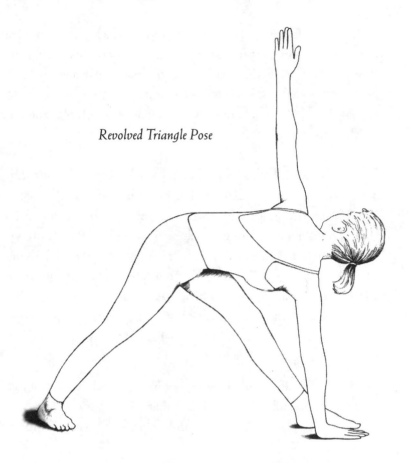

Revolved Triangle Pose

MAKE IT EASIER: If you're pregnant or simply uncomfortable in the pose, use a sturdy chair placed against a wall to get the benefits of this pose. Place your left foot on the chair. Now twist to your left, looking around behind you in that direction. Place your hands where they fall, or reach them out to hold the pose. Repeat on the other side.

SIDE ANGLE TWIST POSE (*Parivritta Parshvakonasana*)

Proceed as in the Revolved Triangle Pose, only intentionally bend the knee you will be bending toward.

Stand with legs wide, arms out to the sides at shoulder height. Turn your left leg out 90 degrees and your right leg in 45 degrees. Bend your left knee to bring your thigh no lower than parallel to the floor. Inhale and stretch wide, fingertip to fingertip. Exhale and revolve this horizontal line around to the left so that your right arm arrives over your left foot. Inhale; radiate outward from your navel center. Exhale; bend from your hips to reach your right hand to the inside or outside of your left foot. If it doesn't get there, place your right hand or elbow on your left thigh. Breathe and continue to twist and radiate. Hold to your comfortable capacity. Twist farther as you exhale, and expand out from your center as you inhale. Inhale to untwist, extend your left leg, and come up. Repeat on the other side.

HALF SPINAL TWIST POSE (*Ardha Matsyendrasana*)

Sit tall with your legs extended in front. Bend your left knee and place your left foot on the floor at the outside of your right knee. Inhale and press down through your sitting bones to elongate your spine and raise your arms overhead. Exhale and twist to the left, lowering your arms. Grab hold of your left knee with your right hand. Place your left hand on the floor a few inches behind your left hip. Turn your head to the back and press gently into the twist. To release from the pose, inhale to raise your arms overhead while turning your torso and head to the front. Exhale with your arms down and extend your bent leg. Repeat on the other side.

MAKE IT EASIER: Sit tall with your legs crossed. Inhale, elongate your spine, and raise your arms overhead. Exhale and twist to the left, letting your arms come down. Place your right hand on your left knee or thigh and your fin-

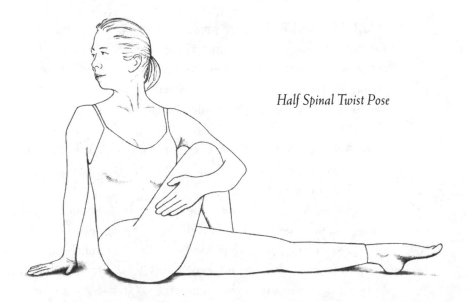

Half Spinal Twist Pose

gertips or palm of your left hand on the floor behind you. Look behind. To release from the pose, inhale and raise your arms overhead while turning to face the front. Exhale and lower your arms. Repeat on the other side with the opposite foot on top.

CHALLENGE ME: For a more intense stretch for the upper back and shoulders, instead of holding your left knee, reach your right arm OVER your left outer thigh and grasp your left ankle from the small toe side.

A FURTHER CHALLENGE: Spinal Twist Pose (*Matsyendrasana*)

Sit tall with your legs extended in front. Bend your right knee, and rotate your leg outward to place your heel at your groin. Bend your left knee and place your foot on the floor outside your right knee. Inhale and raise your arms overhead. Exhale and twist to the left to bring your right elbow to the outside of your left thigh. Wrap your left arm around your back toward your right hip. See if you can deepen the twist to bring your right hand back under your left thigh to clasp your left hand! If you haven't called 911 yet, look back over your left shoulder.

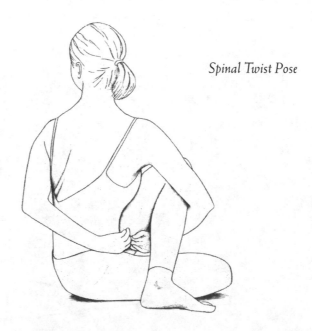

Spinal Twist Pose

Category 7. Hip Mobility and Forward-Bending Poses

A popular Hatha Yoga teacher once quipped that you could reduce all of contemporary Hatha Yoga to the length of the hamstring muscles. As in most jokes, this contains an element of truth. The length of the hamstrings greatly affects our ability to perform many yoga postures and to enjoy ease in the movements of our daily lives. Another key region is the hip area. Being able to move freely through the hips gives you agility, balance, grace, and ease. You are much less likely to get injured during any movement when you have free range of motion in the hips. Picture someone walking with freedom through the hips. What do you see? Youthfulness, sexiness, liveliness, musicality? Now picture someone walking with tight, stiff, hard-to-move hips. What do you see now? Pain? Inhibition? Tension?

It comes as no surprise that the hamstrings and pelvis muscles have their part to play in forward folding. "You are as young as your spine is flexible," my first yoga teacher used to say. Forward folding is difficult for strong protective back muscless and spines stiff from desk jobs. To fold, or rather enfold, into ourselves is to return to a sense of safe withdrawal and release from attending to the world and the needs of those around us. If these poses are difficult at first, please be patient. Recognize and perhaps applaud your strength. Recuperation through forward bending will in the end serve to make you stronger.

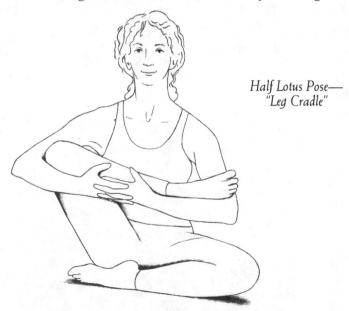

Half Lotus Pose—
"Leg Cradle"

Hip Mobility

HALF LOTUS POSE (*Ardha Padmasana*)–"LEG CRADLE"

Many consider the Lotus Pose to be the domain of only accomplished yoga practitioners. We will use one aspect of this posture for our purpose of hip opening. Sit cross-legged with your spine as erect as possible. Cup your hands underneath your top ankle to gently lift this bent leg off the lower one. Continue to sit erectly by pressing downward through the sitting bones. You can also hold this upper leg by placing your foot in the crook of your nearby elbow and your knee in the crook of your other elbow. Clasp your hands along the outside of your lifted shin. This makes a "leg cradle." Gently rock side to side to soften your pelvis and hips throughout. Then gently lift your leg closer to your chest; sit tall. Repeat on the other side.

BOUND ANGLE POSE (*Baddha Konasana*)

Sit with the soles of your feet together, knees rotated outward. Inhale and reach your arms overhead, elongating your torso. Exhale and bend forward from your hips, bringing your arms down to the floor in front of your body. Breathe and let your head relax toward the floor.

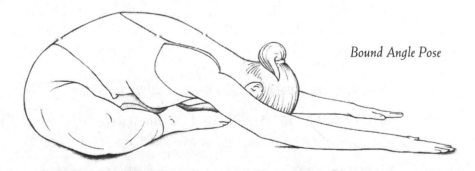

Bound Angle Pose

bizarre fun-to-try tip

There are reflexive patterns through the legs that help deepen this pose. Stimulate the small toe of the foot that you will hold for the "Leg Cradle" by pinching it firmly. Lead with this toe to rotate your leg into the Half Lotus Pose. When you activate this nervous system support, it will allow your leg to fold and rotate more easily into position.

Caution: Use caution with the Bound Angle Pose if you have back problems.

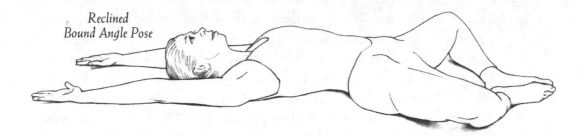

Reclined Bound Angle Pose

CHALLENGE ME: Reclined Bound Angle Pose (*Supta Baddha Konasana*)

THE POWER OF THE POSE: Along with providing hip opening, this pose helps relax tension throughout the pelvis region, allowing organs and glands to operate effectively. It supports the downward flow of *prana* in the lower torso.

Begin as above. Inhale and raise your arms overhead. Exhale and lower your arms behind your back, fingertips at the sides of your pelvis. Slowly lean back onto your elbows. If this works out, continue onto your back. There will be an arch in your lower back. Stretch your arms overhead along the floor. Reverse the process to come up.

SYMBOL OF YOGA POSE (*Yoga Mudrasana*)

THE POWER OF THE POSE: In addition to hip opening, this pose stimulates the ovaries and their glandular function.

VERSION 1: Sit on your heels; make fists. Place them on your thighs at the crease of your hips over your inner thighs. Inhale and then exhale, bending forward over the fists. You want to feel gentle pressure into your abdomen from the placement of your fists. Breathe and relax.

Caution: Do not do the Symbol of Yoga during pregnancy.

VERSION 2: Sit with legs crossed; make fists. Place them above your inner thighs and bend forward. You want to feel gentle pressure through your fists. If you can't bend forward far enough for this effect, use version 1.

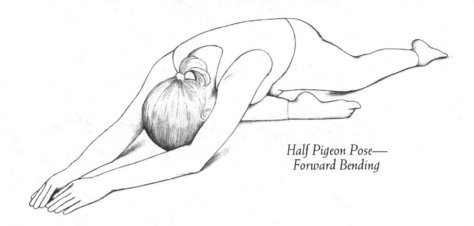

Half Pigeon Pose—
Forward Bending

HALF PIGEON POSE (*Ardha Kapotasana*)– FORWARD BENDING

The Half Pigeon is quite useful for stretching important muscles in your pelvis. Sit on your heels. Allow your pelvis to shift off to the left so your left heel is at your groin. Extend your right leg directly behind you and, if possible, rotate your kneecap toward the floor. Raise your arms overhead and, as you exhale, bend forward from your hip. Allow your head and arms to come to the floor. The left sitting bone should remain on the floor. If you would like to feel a deeper stretch, bring your left heel and shinbone forward. Gently press your chest down onto your shin. If you have a lot of flexibility in the deep rotators of your pelvis, then you'll need to bring your shinbone under your throat and rest your whole torso on the floor. Relax into the pose. When you're ready to come up, inhale with your arms overhead, extending through your spine. Exhale and lower your arms. Repeat on the other side.

HALF HERO POSE (*Ardha Virasana*)

THE POWER OF THE POSE: Along with stretching the thighs, hips, and groin region, the Hero poses also aid in digestion and elimination and in the downward flow of *prana*.

Caution: Use caution with the Half Hero Pose if you have knee problems. Use the *Make It Easier* suggestion and attempt only the first variation.

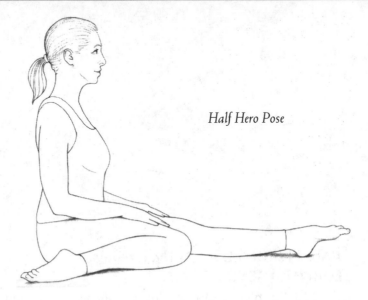

Half Hero Pose

We are using the pose for inward rotation of the thigh in the hip, but this pose naturally involves much more of you than one piece. In preparation, sit with your knees bent, with the soles of your feet on the floor. You can put your hands down behind you for stability if you like. Now rotate your left leg inward so the inside of your left knee aims toward the floor. You may need to rotate your right leg outward at the same time. Repeat this motion easily, moving slowly (don't flop the legs) from side to side several times. This may be enough.

Next, with your left leg rotated inward, extend your right leg out along the floor in front of you. If this feels okay so far, see if you can easily bring the heel of your left foot against your hip, toes pointing back. Your knee may or may not reach the floor. Press your sitting bones into the floor to elongate upward through your spine. Sit tall. Relax and breathe. Do the other side.

MAKE IT EASIER: Sit on a folded towel or blanket to elevate your pelvis.

CHALLENGE ME: Reclined Half Hero Pose (*Ardha Supta Virasana*). To recline this pose, turn your torso toward the extended leg side (left). Tilt over to rest some weight on your elbow, which you can place somewhere near your hip. This may be enough. If your body wants to go farther (not your will, not your sense of adventure—your body), roll backward onto your back. Your lower back will arch off the floor. Breathe and relax. If you feel pain in your knee, get out of the pose. To come out, reverse what you did to get there: Reach your right arm across to the left, and roll toward the left. Roll to the side and then forward to bring you up to sitting.

HERO POSE (*Virasana*)

If the Half Hero Pose is easy for you and you feel absolutely no pain in your knees, try the full Hero Pose. Begin on your hands and knees, with your lower legs rotated slightly inward. SLOWLY sit back between your heels. Your feet can be in tight to your body or turned out to the sides.

CHALLENGE ME: You may want to investigate going to your back from this position into the Reclined Hero Pose (*Supta Virasana*). Put your hands behind your toes, or hold your toes and slowly arch your back to place weight on your elbows. If this seems okay, continue to place your upper back and head on the floor. Yes, this is also a back-bending pose! Extend your arms overhead, palms together. Coming out of the pose is easily accomplished by turning your upper

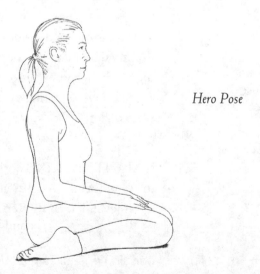

Hero Pose

Caution: Do not do the Hero Pose if you have knee problems.

torso to one side and freeing your foot on the opposite side. Proceed to roll to the side to sit up. You will not strain your thighs, lower back, or knees if you come out of the pose this way.

Forward-Bending Poses

STANDING FORWARD FOLD POSE (*Uttanasana*)

THE POWER OF THE POSE: Soothes the nervous system; releases spinal nerves; tones liver, spleen, and kidneys; stretches back and backs of legs; relaxes neck tension.

From standing, inhale, raise your arms overhead, and elongate your spine. Exhale, bend forward from your hips, and aim the top of your head toward the floor. If you feel an intense pull in your hamstrings, just bend your knees as needed. Allow your head to dangle as if you are rinsing shampoo off the hair at the nape of your neck. If it's uncomfortable to allow your spine and head to hang, bend your knees and place either your hands or your elbows on your thighs. Relax here as long as you're comfortable. Slowly roll up or inhale and extend your spine, bringing your arms out to the sides. For support, curl your tailbone slightly under and elongate through your lower back, knitting together your abdominals in the front. To add more work, bring your arms overhead as you come up. Be sure to extend along your spine in a long flat line as you rise. Exhale and lower your arms.

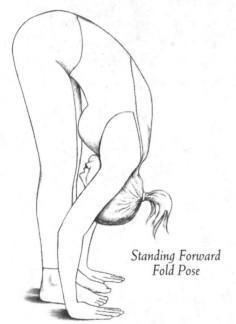

Standing Forward Fold Pose

MAKE IT EASIER: Another way to ease into this pose is to stand facing a wall and place your hands on it at about chest level. Carefully step back, bending over at your hips

Caution: For all forward-bending poses, use caution if you have a disc problem, abdominal problems, sciatica, or high blood pressure. Use support and limit folding to avoid any pelvic compression during pregnancy.

and keeping your hands on the wall. You control how far back you go and how much bend you want.

CHALLENGE ME: (Hold the) Big Toe Pose (*Padangusthasana*)

THE POWER OF THE POSE: Soothes the nervous system; releases the spinal nerves; tones the liver, spleen, and kidneys; stretches the back and the backs of legs; relaxes neck tension.

If forward bending with your legs extended is easy, then complete your folded position by holding onto the big toe of each foot when you arrive. Then lift your upper spine and look forward as you inhale; lower it as you exhale for three or more times. Then hold the fully folded pose, bringing your elbows out to the sides and your forehead to touch your legs. Put your body weight into the pads of your feet, not your heels.

A FURTHER CHALLENGE: If you love this one (I do too!), try it with your hands placed under your feet. Now the posture is called the Hand-to-Foot Pose (*Padahastasana*).

ANGLE POSE (*Konasana*)

THE POWER OF THE POSE: Soothes the nervous system; releases the spinal nerves; tones the liver, spleen, and kidneys; stretches the back and the backs of legs; relaxes neck tension; provides targeted intense stretch to the hamstrings.

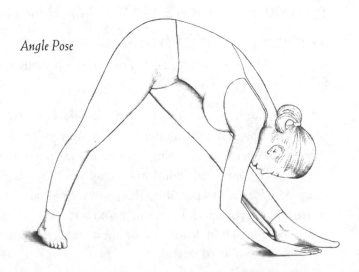

Angle Pose

This variation requires only a slight step forward with one foot, bringing the heel only to the instep and continuing to bend forward. The idea is to purposely put the body into asymmetry so as to release all those knotty spots that remain hidden to our perception when the body works from symmetrical positions. If you find value here, soften your knees to step a little farther out. Breathe and relax. Then step a little farther again, and again. You will want to turn your back foot outward slightly, between 30 and 45 degrees, for better balance as you step farther apart. After bending over in these variations for some time, bend your knees to round up through your back so you can keep the muscles you have just lengthened long as you come up. Then let your other leg take the forward-stepping journey.

MAKE IT EASIER: Sometimes as you bend forward, you reach that place where your hamstring is no longer a happy camper. At this point, simply allow your front knee to bend as much as needed. This is *not* cheating! It is staying within your capacity. Intend (think/feel) length and extension through your entire leg. The extended position will come if you don't force it.

CHALLENGE ME: This will take you into more of a whole body pose than a focus on the lower body. Clasp your hands behind your back. As you fold forward from your hip, lift your hands upward behind your back. You must continue to lengthen through your entire spine by reaching out from your head so as not to round over as your arms lift behind your back. Open your chest.

POSTERIOR STRETCH POSE (*Paschimottanasana*)

THE POWER OF THE POSE: Besides providing a stretch for the entire back of the body (the west side), this posture is especially good for the heart, the abdominal organs, and the pelvic glands.

Sit with your legs extended in front. Inhale and raise your arms overhead, pressing through the sitting bones to extend your spine. Exhale and bend forward from your hips, reaching over your legs. Keep your head between your arms. Place your hands comfortably on your legs, the backs of your knees extended as much as possible. Keep stretching out through the top of your head, making your neck long. Once you find a good stretch here, you may allow your chin to fold down to your chest and your body to droop, letting your elbows soften toward the floor.

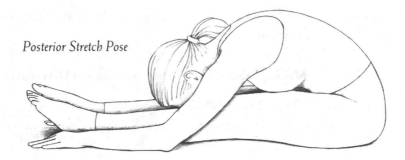

Posterior Stretch Pose

MAKE IT EASIER: You certainly can allow your knees to bend to make this posture possible. A gentle way to do it is *vinyasa krama* style. Sit as before, inhale, and raise your arms overhead. Exhale and bend forward from your hips. Inhale and lengthen upward, leading with your head and arms. Exhale, again bending over and reaching long. Inhale and lengthen up. Repeat this pattern two or more times. This will loosen up the muscles, connective tissues, and organs involved in the pose. When you're ready, once again exhale and lengthen over your legs. See if you can hold the pose more comfortably.

You can also rest your torso on a support, such as a pillow or a folded blanket placed on your thighs, but be sure it's not so large as to prevent you from stretching.

CHALLENGE ME: If this posture is easy when you fold forward, grasp your large toes with your index and middle fingers and thumbs. Flatten your chest

guiding principle: will and surrender

Mystical traditions point out the paradoxical nature of life. Because yoga practice is a virtual practice field for living, it reflects life's inherent contradictions. The dialogue between effort and release, pointed intention and utter detachment, is never more available to us than in yoga postures. They require us to reach at the same time as we yield. Just like the various situations in life, some postures require more will, while others require more surrender. Some must be met with measured alternating current, while still others need an articulate balance of contrasting energies. Forward-bending poses are an excellent way to study this dialogue without strain.

onto your thighs. Look out over your feet and bring your elbows to the floor on the outsides of your legs.

HEAD-TO-KNEE POSE (*Janu Shirshasana*)—FORWARD

THE POWER OF THE POSE: Stretches hamstring muscles, increases flexibility in hip joints and spine, improves circulation, tones spinal nerves, and benefits abdominal organs.

Sit with both legs extended in front of your body. Bend your right knee to rotate your leg out. Place the sole of your right foot against your left inner thigh. Inhale, raise your arms overhead, and stretch your torso. With your spine long, exhale to bend at your hip as far forward as comfortable, keeping your head between your arms. When you feel a stretch in the back of your extended leg, bring your arms to the floor or to your leg. Allow your chin to go into your chest and let your body droop over.

MAKE IT EASIER: If this posture is difficult, change it to a moving loop (*vinyasa krama*). Inhale and reach your arms overhead. Exhale and reach forward along your extended leg. Inhale and lengthen up, leading with your head and arms. Exhale, bend forward and down. Inhale up and exhale over several times; then switch legs.

CHALLENGE ME: As you exhale to reach forward, grasp the sole of your flexed foot with both hands. Bring your chest onto your thigh. Look forward and bring your elbows to the floor. Hold to your comfortable capacity. To come up, stretch your arms out along the floor and lead with your head and arms. Repeat on the other side.

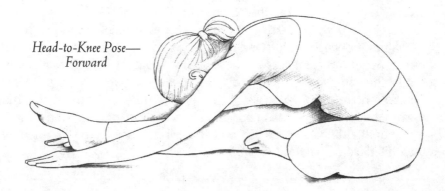

Head-to-Knee Pose— Forward

WIND-ELIMINATING POSE (*Supta Pavanamuktasana*)

THE POWER OF THE POSE: Gently relaxes hip flexor muscles, tones colon, and relieves gas.

Lie supine; bend your left knee and wrap your hands or arms around it. Exhale to gently press your thigh into your torso. Inhale to slowly release. If your neck is not tight or injured, roll your chin to your chest as you exhale and press. Repeat several times.

CHALLENGE ME: Begin with either hands or arms wrapped around both knees. As you exhale, press both knees into your torso. Inhale to release. Repeat several times.

SINGLE-LEG LIFT POSE (*Utthita Ekapadasana*)

THE POWER OF THE POSE: Increases hip flexibility and stretches the legs!

Sit with your right leg turned out, knee bent, heel to your groin. Bend your left leg and hold on to your foot, shin, or just the fabric of your pant leg. Tilt back a bit and extend this leg upward while holding on. You have lots

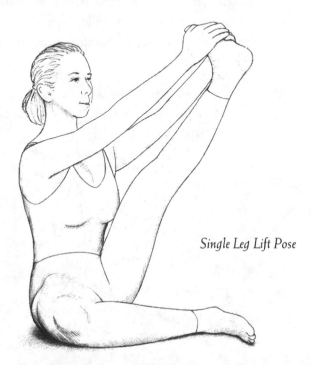

Single Leg Lift Pose

of options here. To intensify the stretch, decrease the angle at your hip. To involve different muscle fibers, cross your extended leg over your body's midline, or open it a bit to the side. Find different muscles that need help and arrange the posture so they can release. Repeat with your other leg.

SPREAD LEG POSE (*Upavishtha Konasana*)

THE POWER OF THE POSE: Improves circulation to pelvis, stretches hips and inner thighs, and stimulates the ovaries.

Sit with your legs apart, kneecaps and toes pointing toward the ceiling. This may be enough! If this is a challenge, place your palms or fingertips on the floor behind you. Work to sit so you feel your sitting bones underneath you rather than having your pelvis tilt back onto the fleshy part.

If you want to try folding forward, inhale first to elongate your spine. Exhale, bring your hands in front of you, and bend forward from your hips. Walk your hands forward. Feel your legs rotate in your hip joints. When you find the edge of the stretch, keep your hands where they are. Breathe slowly and focus on the feeling of the stretch. To come out, curl your tailbone under and gently pull your abdominal muscles in. Walk the hands back and sit up. If you have been in the pose for a while, use your hands to draw your legs together, one at a time, so as not to immediately shorten the muscles you just stretched.

Spread Leg Pose

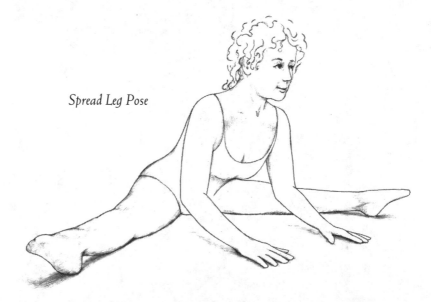

CHALLENGE ME: With experience and practice, you'll eventually be able to rest your belly, chest, and chin on the floor. When this becomes easy (easy?), you can increase the hip stretch by bringing the elbows under the knees. This becomes the Tortoise Pose (*Kurmasana*).

CHILD'S POSE *(Balasana)*

THE POWER OF THE POSE: Relieves minor low back pain and tension, takes pressure off discs through mild natural traction, and reduces sensory stimulation.

Sit on your heels and fold forward from your hips. Your forehead may touch the floor. Adapt this pose to suit you by opening your legs or lifting your pelvis higher. If this pose bothers your knees, roll onto your back and hug your bent legs into your torso. Hold your legs around your thighs (not your shins) to keep from putting pressure on your knees.

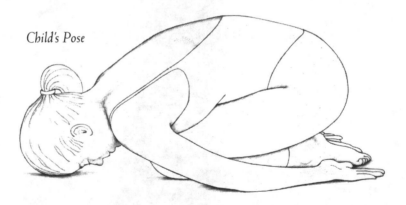

Child's Pose

Caution: Use caution with the Child's Pose if you have knee problems.

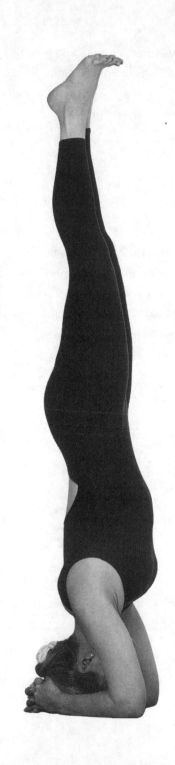

chapter 5

the essential postures for women III
inverted and relaxation poses

Don't go outside your house to see the flowers. My friend, don't bother with that excursion. Inside your body there are flowers. One flower has a thousand petals. That will do for a place to sit. Sitting there you will have a glimpse of beauty.
—Kabir

In the light of calm and steady self-awareness, inner energies wake up and work miracles without any effort on your part.
—Nisargadatta Maharaj

After having worked your way through the fundamental poses in chapters 3 and 4, you are now ready for the more challenging inverted poses and the tranquility of the relaxation poses. Enjoy!

Category 8. Inverted Poses

Inverted poses are tricky. You need their benefit most when you shouldn't be doing them. Similar to the twisting poses, but with even more bang for the buck, inverted postures affect your entire body and all its systems and tissues. These practices intensely alter the currents of *prana* in your body. You do not want to overwhelm an area that may already be struggling. You could considerably worsen your existing condition so please pay close attention to the cautions. To make inverted poses easier, I've included the Legs on Chair alternative. It's safe for everyone who can lie comfortably on the floor, and you accrue many of the benefits of inverting, particularly the fluid drainage from the lower extremities.

THE POWER OF INVERTED POSES: Balances and revitalizes all body systems; aids in tissue regeneration; encourages diaphragmatic breathing; improves blood flow to the head, brain, eyes, and ears; helps in preventing neck ailments. Tones nerves and calms the mind; counters normal orientation in the field of gravity and thus changes fluid flows, drains blood and lymph from lower limbs, revitalizes brain, replenishes organs. Regulates thymus, pituitary, pineal, thyroid and parathyroid glands, and carotid and mammillary bodies.

SPREAD LEG FORWARD FOLD POSE (*Prasarita Padottanasana*)
Stand with your legs wide, toes pointing forward. Inhale and raise your arms to the sides at shoulder height. Exhale and bend forward from your hips, keep-

Caution for ALL Inverted Poses: Do not do these poses if you have fever, headache, head injury, glaucoma, or eye pressure issues. Do not do if you have heart disease, high blood pressure, thrombosis, or enlarged liver or spleen. Do not do if you have disc problems. I feel it is best to avoid true inversions (not just putting your feet up, which *is* recommended) during menses and after the third month of pregnancy.

guiding principle: how far for how long?

Your body-mind's edges are the guides to how deeply you go into a pose and how long you hold it. Some people like numbers. Holding a pose for three long steady breaths is usually a good minimum. I feel it takes our nervous system that long to settle into what we're doing. If we're comfortable enough to stay longer, we can then enter into further dialogue with our tensions. Any stretch should feel good when it's over, even if you feel a lot of intensity while it's happening. You should never feel joint pain at any point during or after a pose or posture sequence, because this means something is wrong, possibly with your alignment.

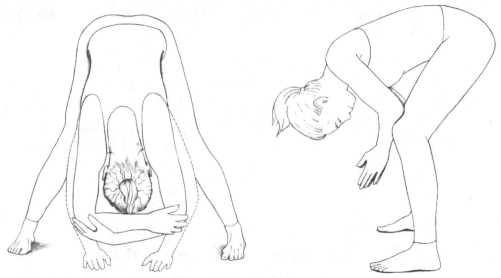

Spread Leg Forward Fold   *Spread Leg Forward Fold—Make it Easier*

ing your knees slightly bent so energy can run through them. Do what you want with your arms or hold your opposite elbow. Also try reaching them through your legs, putting the backs of your hands on the floor. Relax here as long as you are comfortable. To come up, curl your tailbone slightly under and elongate through your lower back as you inhale, bringing your arms out to the sides. As you find your whole body integration to do this (as in category 2 practices), add more work by bringing your arms overhead as you come up. Lengthen along your spine as you rise. Exhale and lower your arms.

MAKE IT EASIER: Do either or both of the following:

1. If this is too much of an intense stretch for your hamstrings, bend your knees.

2. If it is uncomfortable to allow your spine and head to hang, bend your knees and place either your hands or elbows on your thighs. Round your back to come up.

INVERTED ACTION POSE (*Viparita Karani*)

VERSION 1: Lie supine, with your arms next to your body. Exhale and bend your knees to draw your thighs into your torso. Inhale and extend your legs upward. Exhale, push with your arms, and roll your pelvis off the floor, with your legs going over your upper torso and head. Bend your arms to place your hands on your hips, which will be above your elbows. This may be enough!

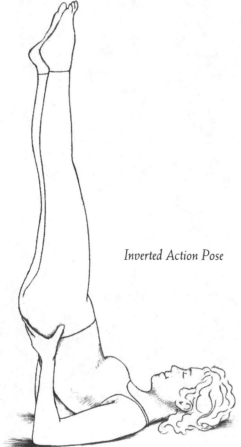

Inverted Action Pose

VERSION 2: If you've decided to lift your legs upward to a more vertical position, check to see that your elbows are in line with your shoulders, not way out to the sides. Ready? Inhale and raise your legs perpendicular to the floor. Ta-daa! Breathe evenly and hold to your comfortable capacity.

This posture is so good for you that it is worth trying to extend the amount of time you spend in it. Begin with twenty to thirty seconds. (You may find it helpful to use a kitchen timer.) Stay longer by adding on small increments of twenty to thirty seconds. Some of our classes work up to holding this pose in class for ten minutes.

CHALLENGE ME: Shoulder Stand Pose (*Sarvangasana*)

THE POWER OF THE POSE: In addition to the benefits of inverting, this pose strengthens the arms, chest, shoulders, back, and abdomen and stretches the back of the neck while compressing the front of the neck to further stimulate the thymus, in particular improving immune support. Improves blood flow focused on the neck, and improves blood flow to the head, brain, eyes, and ears.

Caution: Beyond the other cautions for inverted poses, do not do this pose if you have neck problems. This may sound silly, but come down if you need to cough, yawn, or sneeze.

Go through version 1 of the Inverted Action Pose (*Viparita Karani*). Bend your elbows and place your hands on your back, fingers pointing inward. Place them as far down near your shoulders as possible. This will allow you to straighten upward from your upper spine. Press down on your elbows to raise your extended legs, allowing your pelvis to move slightly forward in line with your legs. Press your breastbone toward your chin. Breathe evenly.

You can feel the weight of your abdominal organs on your diaphragm muscle as you breathe in the posture. You are giving them a wonderful massage and allowing the more stagnant blood that pools in their lower portions a chance to circulate.

SUPPORTED INVERSION POSES

Here are some gentle alternatives to the free-standing inverted postures.

VERSION 1: Legs on Chair. Sit sideways, just in front of a chair. Tilt away from the chair onto your side and then roll onto your back. As you do, lift your bent legs up onto the chair and rest your lower legs on it. Rest here as long as you like. Come out of the pose by reversing this process.

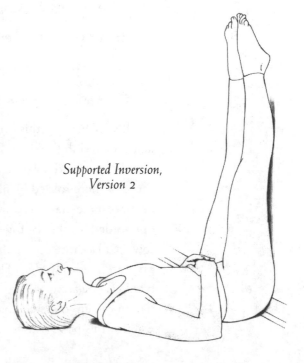

Supported Inversion, Version 2

VERSION 2: Feet up Wall. Sit near but not quite touching a wall or locked door, face sideways. Tilt away from the wall onto your side and then roll onto your back. As you do, lift your bent legs up. Extend your legs up the wall, hands on your abdomen, palms down. Or exhale to press into the floor with your arms and into the wall with your feet. Slowly increase the bend of your knees as you lift your pelvis off the floor. If this feels fine, you may experiment with lifting one leg at a time off the wall. Come out of the pose by reversing this process.

VERSION 3: The Perfect Wedge. This is a gentle alternative to shoulder-standing postures because it benefits you without as much work. There are a number of ways to use props to suit your particular body proportions. A rectangular-shaped bolster comes in handy, but if you collect enough blankets from your cold weather storage, you can make them work.

Sometimes when we do this pose in class, we have an erector set moment when everyone gets different combinations of bolsters, pillows, small soft balls, blankets, and their own clothing to construct "the perfect wedge" for this pose. Here is a basic setup, but use it as a beginning guideline. If you build a better mousetrap for this pose, you will be so outrageously comfortable that you'll stay and stay and stay!

You might want to use:

❋ A rectangular-shaped bolster (a round one is higher if you are tall)

❋ 4 to 6 blankets, the denser the fabric the better

❋ 2 to 6 bath towels

❋ A sticky mat to keep things from sliding away from the wall

If you're doing this on an uncarpeted floor, you may want to put a sticky mat down, with the short side against the wall. This can keep everything from sliding apart and away from the wall when you get on. Place the bolster or three or more folded blankets with the long side against the wall. Place two or three more blankets or large folded beach towels next to the first pile. Place one folded blanket or towel next to that. You may want to roll up two beach towels. Place one on top of the lowest step and one on top of the second lowest step of your wedge. This will give you more of a wedge than steps if the blankets you are using are very firm. Experiment wildly. I know someone who has an old upholstered chair that she turns upside down and puts against her wall for this pose (I'm not making this up!). If you want something more elegant, Larry Jacobs, an expert on inverting the body for health, has devised an inversion wedge called the Body Slant. See appendix D.

PLOW POSE *(Halasana)*

THE POWER OF THE POSE: This is one of the most rejuvenating of all postures! The pressure of the breath in this pose massages internal organs, improving spleen, pancreas, liver, and kidney functions. It increases flexibility in the spine, upper back, and neck; regulates the thyroid and suprarenal glands; and promotes insulin production by stimulating the pancreas. It also stimulates the thymus, improving immune response; tones spinal nerves; and activates digestion.

Lie supine, with your knees bent and the soles of your feet on the floor. Draw your knees into your chest, extend your legs, and roll your pelvis off the floor. Allow your legs to extend beyond your head. If this pose is easy, allow your feet to touch the floor beyond your head, rolling your toes under. Breathe evenly and remain there as long as you like. If this still feels good, you may walk your feet away from your head until your chin is against your chest. Use your abdominal muscles and your hands at your sides against the floor to slowly roll down.

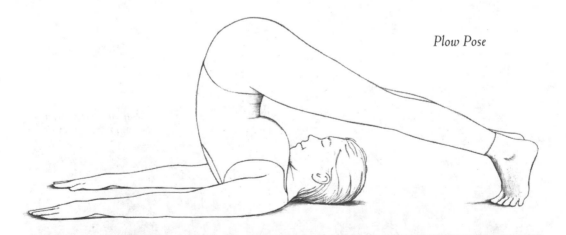

Plow Pose

Caution: Beyond the inverted cautions above, do not do the Plow Pose if you have a hernia, high blood pressure, serious back or neck problems, slipped disc, or sciatica.

DOLPHIN POSE, PREPARATION FOR SCORPION POSE
(Vrishchikasana)

THE POWER OF THE POSE: The Dolphin and Scorpion Poses are advanced postures that require a great deal of perseverance, hand and upper-body strength, balance, and, most significantly, fearlessness. The Dolphin helps develop the upper body stability for the other pose. More than the physical benefits of opening the chest and inverting, these postures reduce the grasp of the ego. In the Scorpion, I feel as though my yoga practice is dangling me over a cliff and shaking me free of all my ego investments. When it's over, it's really quite refreshing!

There are several inverted poses that require balance on the forearms. A good way to prepare for these postures is to work in the upper body position without taking the feet off the ground. Sometimes this preparatory position is called the Dolphin Pose.

Begin on your hands and knees with your hips over your knees and your hands slightly forward of your shoulders. Lower your forearms to the floor, keeping them parallel. Lift your pelvis up through your sitting bones while extending your legs. Aim the top of your head toward the floor. If you can keep

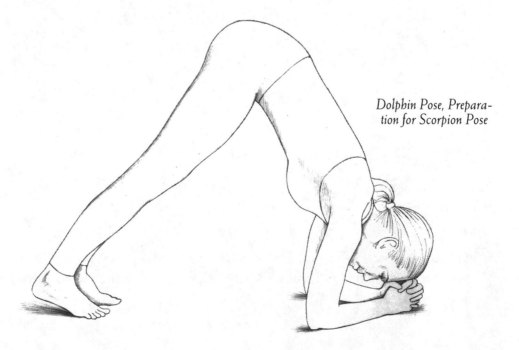

Dolphin Pose, Preparation for Scorpion Pose

your elbows pressing into the floor without collapsing through your spine, then you may lift your head up so your face is parallel to the floor.

CHALLENGE ME: Scorpion Pose (*Vrishchikasana*).

From the Dolphin Pose, lift your right leg up as high as you can toward vertical. Press down through your forearms and push off with your left foot. Use as little "umph" as possible so you don't overshoot or collapse through your chest and upper spine. Carefully arch your spine and allow your knees to bend over your head. Here you have the added benefit of a balance challenge in a mega-strengthening inverted position.

HEAD STAND POSE (*Shirshasana*)

Learned opinion varies greatly on the appropriateness of this pose for "non-adepts." Some teachers hold off on this practice until the advanced-level course. Others introduce it to senior beginners in the winter without a warm-up (I've seen it!). Even though you may not have any serious counterindications to prevent you from doing this pose, be mindful of days when your neck is stiff, you are traveling, or you had a bad night. Make sure your upper torso is warmed up sufficiently, and don't do it if you're tired or absent-minded . . . please! There's always tomorrow.

Sit on your heels, lean forward, then clasp your hands and place them and your forearms on the floor in front of you. Your elbows should be a forearm's length apart. Place the hairline of your forehead on the floor between your forearms, about four inches from your hands. Raise your hips by extending your legs while you roll onto the top of your head. Walk your feet toward your face a few steps, bringing your pelvis higher. This will give you many of the benefits of this pose, so feel free to stop now.

Be sure to press down through your elbows, forearms, and edges of your hands. As you do, slowly draw both bent legs off the floor. This is a great basic position for getting used to the feeling of the full headstand. You may wish to practice this for awhile before going further.

Caution: Do not do the Head Stand Pose if you have *any* neck problems.

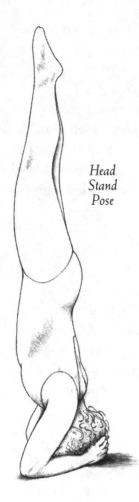

*Head
Stand
Pose*

Next, lift your thighs, keeping your knees bent, and finally, fully extend your legs. Remember to press your forearms into the floor for balance. This is where most of the body weight should be, not on your head. If you feel any pain in your head or neck, or just feel a little funny, come down! This posture is terrific for feeling your diaphragm while you're breathing. Shoot for comfortably staying in the pose for a minute. Reverse the entire process step by step to come down.

After completing the pose, rest a few moments with your head down. Then sit up for a few moments. Then rest on your back.

Category 9. Relaxation Poses

In combination with diaphragmatic breathing, relaxation is a core technique necessary for every posture. In relaxation practice, you learn to search for and release unnecessary tensions. This not only provides you with a transition into and out of practice, and between more challenging sections of your work, but it also gives you an opportunity to practice a central yogic technique. Then as you work your way into the more challenging active poses, you use this very method to efficiently apply only what willpower and physical exertion you need.

Relaxation practice gives you a chance to practice efficient exertion and attend to your body's subtle and sometimes not-so-subtle signals of imbalance. By reducing the noise of activity and drawing attention inward (*pratyahara*), relaxation provides an opening to doing inner work through yoga, as explored later in this book. Learn to release tension in your yoga practice. Then apply the method to the rest of your life! Relaxation practice also allows you to naturally recharge your batteries when you need a break.

SYSTEMATIC RELAXATION

When you're in a chosen relaxation pose, focus first on smooth, even, diaphragmatic breathing. Then focus on each area of your body from head to toes, progressively relaxing each area. Here is a simple order for relaxation:

* ✳ Head and face

* ✳ Neck

* ✳ Upper torso and shoulder area

* ✳ Arms, hands, and fingers

* ✳ Middle torso

* ✳ Lower torso and hips

* ✳ Legs, feet, and toes

Return to paying attention to steady diaphragmatic breathing. A ballpark amount of time for this is ten minutes. The great thing about relaxation is that you can do it all in a few seconds! Just *go* there. Or try this: Relax each of your body areas listed above, taking about eight seconds for each one. You'll get it all in under a minute. When we do this in workshops, a minute seems like a long time. Did it make a difference? Try it in thirty seconds. See, you *do* have time to relax!

BASIC RELAXATION POSE (*Shavasana*)

Lie on your back with your legs spread as wide as your hips or slightly farther apart. Place your arms slightly away from your sides, palms up. You may wish to lift your head off the floor, lengthen it away from your torso, then return it to the floor. Scoop your tailbone under and then let go. Feel symmetrical and evenly spread out throughout your entire body.

MAKE IT EASIER (**more comfortable**): If this position is not comfortable, try bending your knees and placing the soles of your feet on the floor. If your

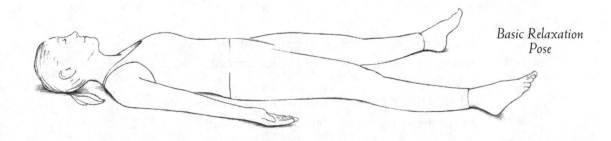

Basic Relaxation Pose

guiding principle:
relaxation and diaphragmatic breathing

One summer weekend, a swami famous for impossible yogic feats was scheduled to teach advanced yoga practices. People excitedly flocked to the yoga center. After years of serious practice, they were going to learn ancient esoteric practices at last! A real yogic feather in the cap and sense of accomplishment prevailed. (If you didn't already see this coming, an exhibition of pride is usually the sign of a setup in spiritual stories.)

On the first day, the famed swami taught relaxation and diaphragmatic breathing. People were a bit put out, but figured that laying the groundwork was necessary. The second day consisted of more relaxation and more detailed attention to the steady motion of the diaphragm. Was this a hoax? The tearoom buzzed with dissension that evening. On the third day, a young man bravely interrupted the swami as he began his lecture—not a small feat, because the swami was a man of great stature and ferocious charisma. The young man urgently inquired whether the swami had planned to teach any of the esoteric practices he had advertised.

Like a lion holding a mouse in its paw, the swami asked, "And which practices are those?"

Now feeling he was getting somewhere, the young man replied, "The ones that enable you to stop your heartbeat and change your skin temperature at will." A hush fell over the auditorium. Everyone strained to hear the response.

"Sir, I AM teaching you THOSE practices," was the reply.

This story illustrates that relaxation is the very essence of Hatha Yoga practice, not an afterthought. Steady diaphragmatic breathing is the bedrock of all of yoga's physical techniques, not just a beginning practice. It is said that if one can master even diaphragmatic breathing, one has accomplished all that yoga has to offer.

hips permit it, turn the heels out and toes in so you can allow your knees to rest against one another. Scoop your tailbone under and then let go.

CROCODILE POSE (Makarasana)

Lie prone with your legs far apart. If you were a crocodile, you would have a very big tail and little legs turned out to the sides. Fold your arms in front and

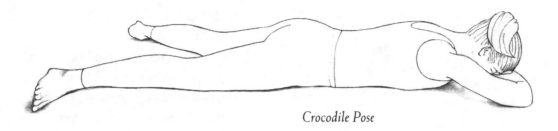

Crocodile Pose

rest your head on your forearms. Relax any effort in your neck and shoulders. If this is difficult, change the arm position to one that feels easy on your neck and shoulders, or turn your head to one side. If it's uncomfortable to turn your legs out, just rotate them in. Let your body's weight sink into the earth. Focus your attention on the motion of the diaphragm.

FLAPPING FISH POSE (*Matsya Kridasana*)

My adult students named this the Serta Mattress Pose, which reflects the level of relaxation it creates. My children students call it the Lizard-on-the-Wall Pose, which interestingly indicates the neurological pattern that would support this position in movement (homolateral body half).

Lie prone and turn your head to the right; bring your right knee up and your right elbow down, so you are partially on your side and partially on your front. You may want to bring your left elbow overhead on the floor so as to put the back of your hand under your cheek. Remain here as long as you like. Try the other side, too!

MAKE IT EVEN EASIER: Use supports to make this pose even more comfortable. For those who are more than a few months into pregnancy, this is one way to be comfy: Place two folded blankets under your bent knee, a pillow under your head, and a rolled blanket or towel under your bent elbow. Rest.

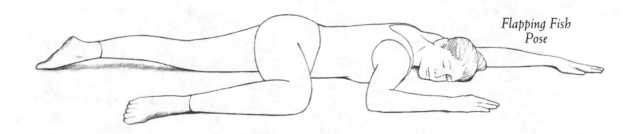

Flapping Fish Pose

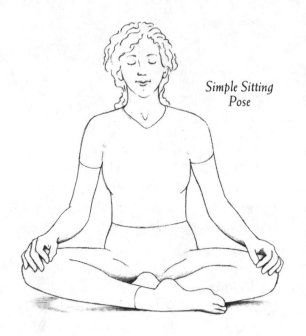

Simple Sitting Pose

SIMPLE SITTING POSE
(*Sukhasana*)

When you picture a meditative posture, you might think of a person sitting bolt upright with her legs tied into a pretzel. Relaxation is a precursor for meditation. While yoga's various folded-leg sitting postures give stability for sitting on the ground, what's important is the erect spine. Practice relaxing in a sitting position by aligning your head, neck, and torso in a chair. On the floor, fold your legs in any comfortable arrangement.

An "at the office mini-practice" could be to check your sitting alignment, breathe deeply, and relax your body from head to toe without any of your co-workers knowing! Practice sitting erectly without extraneous tension. You'll conserve energy, develop greater mental clarity, and reduce muscular tension that develops due to faulty alignment.

SUPPORTED RELAXATION POSE

Using a few props can help you be more comfortable in your relaxation practice, especially when your back and neck muscles are stiff. A simple way to create more ease throughout your body is to roll up two blankets together and place them under your knees before you lie down. You can make a similar roll

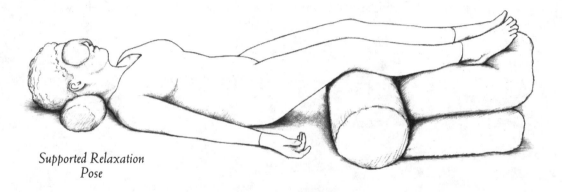

Supported Relaxation Pose

and put it under your feet as well. Have a bath towel nearby and roll it to fit comfortably under the curve of your neck. Don't feel you need to use the entire towel; you can just roll it up part way and let your head rest on the unrolled portion.

Covering your eyes with a warm eye bag or just some soft fabric, such as the sweatshirt you took off earlier, feels great and supports your ability to relax and focus inward. Allow your breath to flow evenly and deeply. Let go!

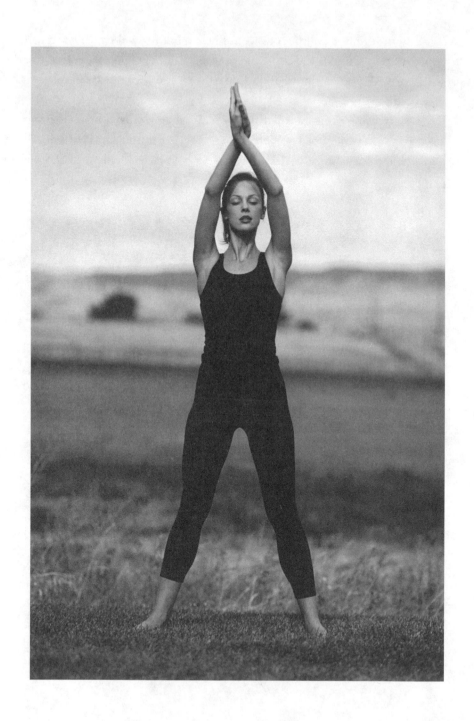

chapter 6

the essential moving practices for women

*Close attention to one's breath, which should synchronize with one's move-
ments, is samapatti (fixing the mind), and breath is the link between mind
and body. . . . While practicing asana, done with purposeful breathing and
fixity of mind, one achieves steadiness and relaxation, which is asana siddhi
(accomplishment in asana). Then one is not affected by the pairs of opposites
. . . such as heat and cold, ridicule and praise, success and failure; his endurance is greatly improved.*

—Srivatsa Ramaswami

*I see the body as being like sand. It's difficult to study the wind; but if you can
watch the way sand patterns form and disappear and re-emerge, then you can
follow the pattern of the wind, or in this case the mind . . . mostly what I observe
is the process of mind.*

—Bonnie Bainbridge Cohen

movement, flow, and health

Movement is a crucial ingredient in vibrant health. Its value as a healing and health-maintaining force is further supported by yoga's sister life-science, *Ayurveda*. For these ancient life-sciences, optimal health is the well-channeled flow of substances and energies into and out of the living being. Physical movement is essential for healthy flow at all levels of existence. Yoga postures and movements route flow along the body's many various channels in very specific ways that support our total well-being.

It may be difficult to recognize movement as a major key to health in our sedentary modern culture. For many of us, any significant movement experience must be planned, purposeful, and compartmentalized. At the end of a chair-bound workday, we emerge from our cubicle, drive to the gym, and wait in line to walk on a treadmill—indoors. Very few of us have lifestyles that require us to work physically for sustenance, as was the case only a generation ago. Even in my lifetime, the forest I grew up playing in—climbing trees, building forts—is far too dangerous (not to mention whittled down and polluted) for my children to explore on their own. Our bodies are a part of nature, and they function best when they move. Our Western penchant for looking at problems piecemeal does not conceive of the widespread lack of venue for physical activity and expression as a major health concern. Occasional studies hit the media stating that people who exercise regularly live longer, but these studies do not embrace the greater value of a life endowed with rich and varied movement experiences.

the integrative state

Movement is a crucial feature of yoga practice as well. Some experts claim that the original discipline of Hatha Yoga was not based on the static postures practiced today, but on movements that constellate around and are thus associated with these postures. They say the static poses were passed down as a short-hand way of indicating rich areas of integrative movement experience.

Most people use the postures to cultivate a healthy body, but we must not forget that the mind and body interact to a much greater extent than Western opinion has acknowledged. Recent scientific findings in the West support what was well known to ancient yoga practitioners in the East: that many diseases are physical manifestations of mental and emotional disturbances. Our physical health is dependent on our emotional and mental well-being and vice versa.

How yoga works has been a burning question for most of my life. I have found that I cannot adequately explain yoga's almost magical potency to someone who doesn't recognize (or experience) the relationship between mind and body, that is, that a physical experience always involves the mind and emotions, and, conversely, that each thought and feeling has an impact on every cell in our body—all the time! Each yoga practice, whether it emphasizes moving, holding a pose, tending the breath, or focusing the mind, invites you to integrate body, breath, mind, and emotions. When you do, you arrive at a psychophysical state of being (notice I'm not saying state of mind) that is unique and specific to that practice. A principal idea in yoga is that the breath is the link between the mind and the body. Different practices bring you into this integrative state by focusing on one, two, or all three of these aspects: body, breath, and mind.

My research on how yoga works took me to teachers who come into this integral state of yoga from different points of entry. Of the many teachings I received from them, I learned that getting in touch with different aspects of my physical body—such as paying attention to my organs, my bones, or my blood—creates within me distinct mental states. I learned that in altering the flow of breath, I could redirect emotions. I learned that the body's tissues themselves express the mind, and this is how some yogis are able to read in a person's face and body carriage every trial and tribulation that person has ever had. I learned that spontaneous movement arising out of the unconscious can reveal important information about a person's angels, demons, ambitions, fears, and the dynamism among them. I learned that poses such as the Turtle or the Cobra or the Tree connect us, through our physicality, to other life-forms that are organized in the same way the poses organize our human body. I learned that the body cannot lie. And I learned (to use a phrase Joseph Campbell used in describing the message of the Holy Grail myth) that spirituality is the bouquet of natural life, not something imposed from above.

archetypes of experience

Yoga postures and yoga movements are two sides of the same coin. The coin is the integrative state of being engendered by the practice. The static poses offer a distillation of experience, a stopover on a journey. They allow us to deeply explore the posture's effect on all levels of our being. Each pose has something unique to offer, for each one will circuit energy through the body in a specific way while activating certain aspects of anatomy and not others.

The experience of the practitioner brought about by the physical constellation of the pose is intentional and a key to understanding how yoga practice works. Some of the names for poses, such as the Hero Pose, reflect the "mind" or "feeling tone" of the pose. If you didn't know what this pose looked like and someone asked you to make it up, you would probably do something that looked heroic and a lot like the classical pose! Some poses, such as the Cobra Pose, are named for animals. The psychophysical state of being represented by the Cobra Pose is a far cry from that of the Hero Pose. When we embody this pose and movements that can be done from it, we activate the parts of our anatomy that bring us into a snake-like consciousness, using the same lower brain patterns that the snake uses in its movement as we locate spinal support and digestive integrity. The power of each posture is often listed as a number of health benefits, but the healing takes place through the total experience of the archetype of the pose: the physical position, the specific channeling of energy, and the frame of mind the pose induces in the practitioner.

yoga movement practice

If holding a pose provides a layover for investigation, then moving practices take you on a journey. In doing them, you may pause, but you don't get off the train. My colleagues and I work with moving practices in two important ways: dynamic postures (*vinyasa krama*) and movement research.

DYNAMIC POSTURES: *VINYASA KRAMA*

Dynamic posture practice, or *vinyasa krama*, is an approach to yoga that uses the breath to thread together various postures. You have seen a few of them already in chapters 3, 4, and 5. Breath and movement patterns can be graceful and connected, or erratic and mentally irritating. When you coordinate movement with breath, your physical effort is streamlined and you are more efficient in what you do. When you practice this coordination regularly, all your actions become more integrated and your attention improves. Dynamic posture practice is useful to warm the body, balance muscular release, lubricate the joints, and soften the connective tissue. Moving practice is often more helpful in releasing chronic muscular tension than are postures that are static. Bodies that are older, out of shape, sedentary (or all three) stand to gain the most benefit.

A dynamic or moving posture can be based on a simple repetitive movement such as bending over and coming up, or lifting a leg and lowering it. This is very useful when a posture is difficult for you to hold for any length of time. A slightly more involved moving practice connects a few postures in a short movement loop. This is my favorite kind of practice because it allows me to focus on my way of supporting the transition between only two or three poses. It is a manageable amount, like a short excursion, so I can focus intently on my alignment and breath support. Dynamic posture practice also includes long, choreographed posture sequences with many postures strung together in a purposeful order.

If you try these practices, you'll probably find that there is much more to explore. If this way of working suits you, see appendix A for suggestions. Here are a few examples of dynamic posture practices you are likely to see in yoga class.

Repetitive Moving Postures

A simple way to approach moving posture practice is to move one part of your body repetitively into and out of a posture while concentrating on the motion of the breath. This could take the form of simply bending over and coming up, lifting and lowering an arm or leg, or extending and bending a knee. This is a very useful approach to posture practice if holding a pose for any length of time is difficult for you. You might be able to repeat the motion eight or nine times, whereas holding the completed posture for even a few seconds may be truly painful. And after you have done the dynamic practice, your body is often prepared to then hold the pose. However, this is not necessarily the aim; the dynamic practices are valuable in their own right.

HEAD-TO-KNEE DYNAMIC POSE
(*Janu Shirshasana Vinyasa Krama*)–FORWARD

Sit with your right leg folded in, heel toward your groin, left leg extended forward. Inhale; raise your arms overhead, stretching throughout the torso. Exhale and keep the extension as you bend forward from your hips, reaching long toward your toes. You may want to bend your knees slightly. Keeping the torso extended, inhale and unfold at the hip and come up. Keep the arms overhead. Repeat four or more times, exhaling over and inhaling up, on each side.

Next try this method with any forward-folding pose, such as the Posterior Stretch Dynamic Pose (*Paschimottanasana Vinyasa Krama*), the Bound Angle Dynamic Pose (*Baddha Konasana Vinyasa Krama*), and Standing Forward Fold Pose (*Uttanasana*). Then try poses from other categories.

Short Posture Loops

This type of breath-coordinated moving practice loops two or a few postures. Shorter sequences such as this one give us a chance to re-pattern correct alignment and support and warm up basic patterns of coordination, if we tune in. When done repeatedly, shorter loops offer a good warm-up for longer sequences and for holding the more challenging postures. Here's a short posture loop that encourages you to integrate your arms and legs with your head and torso:

CHILD'S POSE TO PLANK POSE DYNAMIC PRACTICE
(*Balasana* to *Adho Mukha Dandasana Vinyasa Krama*)

Sit on your heels with your body folded forward, head to the floor. Extend your arms in front of your head, palms on the floor. Inhale and reach forward and up into a hands-and-knees position. Have your hands slightly in front of your shoulders at this point because you'll be going to Plank Pose next. Exhale back to sit on your heels in Child's Pose. Repeat this a few times to get the feel of it. As you do, practice curling your tailbone under and engaging the abdominal wall for low back alignment and support. Slide the shoulder blades low on your back, keeping the shoulders away from the ears and the chest.

Tuck your toes under in Child's Pose. Inhale. This time as you go forward, lift your knees so you come to Downward-Facing Plank Pose, which is the high point of a push-up. (You may need to adjust your hands farther away from your hips, depending on your proportions.) Exhale, round the spine, and sit back on the heels once again. Repeat this as many times as you like, coordinating the breath with the movement. Can you get a good sense of the spine and how it moves when the body is in this arrangement? What else do you notice about the way your body performs this practice?

Long Posture Sequences

The Sun Salutation (*Surya Namaskara*) is a classical sequence used in most popular Western styles of yoga. It's a great warm-up and workout and, when done attentively, develops coordination of breath and movement. Several postures (*asanas*) are connected in this sequence. Additional ones can be stirred in to lengthen the initial sequences. The landmarks are Backward-Bending Pose (*Urdhvasana*), Standing Forward Fold Pose (*Uttanasana*), Monkey Pose (*Banarasana*), Eight-Point Pose (*Ashtanamaskara*), Upward-Facing Dog Pose (*Urdhva Mukha Shvanasana*), and Downward-Facing Dog Pose (*Adho Mukha Shvanasana*).

One aspect that makes this sequence so fascinating is the possibility of breathing in so many different ways with the movements. This aspect of the Sun Salutation keeps me interested in it and able to adapt it to my changing needs, even though I have done the same practice for many years. I suggest you take three deep breaths in each position as you learn it. This is also a good way to go when you're really cold and stiff. When you first learn this sequence, move slowly. Once you know what the positions feel like, try the sequence the way I describe it below. This is a very natural way to do it and is not terribly strenuous. Later, if you want to practice the series at a faster pace, perform two positions on each breath cycle, which means you move as you breathe in and you move to a new position as you breathe out. Begin by breathing in as you arch back.

There are other possibilities I won't describe here. No one way of breathing with this sequence is more correct than the others. They are just different ways that meet different needs. It's far better to match the practice to your body's capacity than to go hurtling over the edge. Less is more.

Adapt as needed! Place a chair to get up from and down to the floor, bend your knees when you need to, and slow it down. Think about how this series can be exactly right for you, then change it to suit you. Improvise new variations no one has ever done before! A good friend gave me a black-and-white print by a famous painter of a woman sitting as if in a yoga twisting pose. It was beautiful, but my apartment at the time was filled with bold secondary colors. The black and white just didn't work. One day, I got the print off the wall and painted three bold lines—purple, turquoise, orange—around the woman's curves. Now it was just right. Here is the Sun Salutation. Make it your own.

SUN SALUTATION (*Surya Namaskara*)

1. Stand tall in Mountain Pose (*Tadasana*); exhale.

2. Inhale. Raise the arms overhead in Standing Staff Pose (*Samasthiti Dandasana*), forearms next to the ears. Exhale and stretch upward.

3. Inhale. Arch backward into the Backward-Bending Pose (*Urdhvasana*). Slightly bend your knees and allow your pelvis to move forward. Extend through your spine. Create a long bow-like curve from the ankles to the top of the head, with the arms still next to the ears. (You'll see this posture done with legs straight and head dangling backward. Our way is spinal-disc friendly.) Exhale.

4. Inhale; extend upward from the base of the skull to standing, arms overhead.

5. Exhale and reach forward, bending at the hips into the Standing Forward Fold Pose (*Uttanasana*). Aim your head toward the floor; your hands may or may not reach it. (This is a great time to stay and breathe.)

6. Inhale. Stretch your right leg back to lunge, placing your right knee and top of your foot on the floor. Look up, or arch up, arms overhead, and balance here in the Monkey Pose (*Banarasana*). (This is another fine place to pause and breathe.)

7. Exhale and bend forward, place your palms on the floor, and lower your body all the way to the floor like

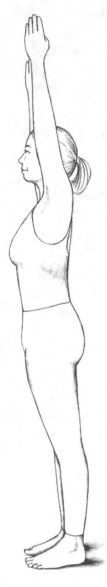

Standing Staff Pose

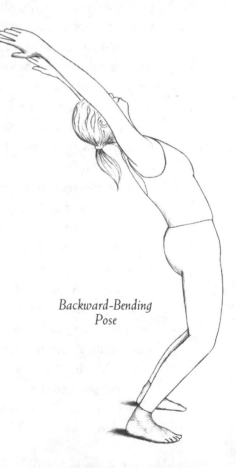

Backward-Bending Pose

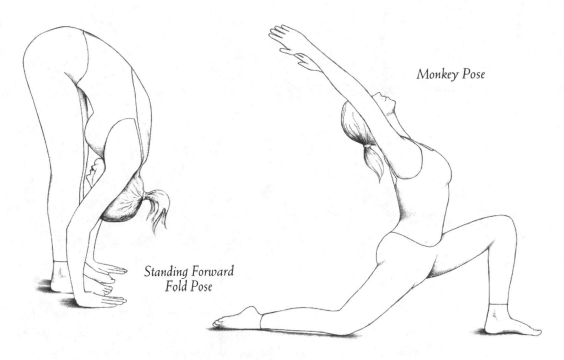

Monkey Pose

*Standing Forward
Fold Pose*

this: Drop the knees, chest, and nose or forehead to the floor for the Eight-Point Pose (*Ashtanamaskara*). Then come in for a landing, moving toward your head.

8. Inhale, lift into a comfortable, well-supported Upward-Facing Dog Pose (*Urdhva Mukha Shvanasana*) by arching the upper body up and back, palms on the floor next to your chest, elbow creases facing one another and slightly bent.

9. Exhale; lower your upper body.

10. Inhale; tuck your toes and get ready to push.

Eight-Point Pose

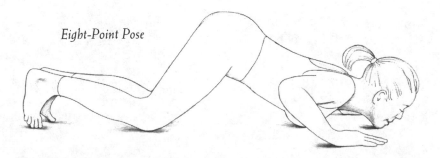

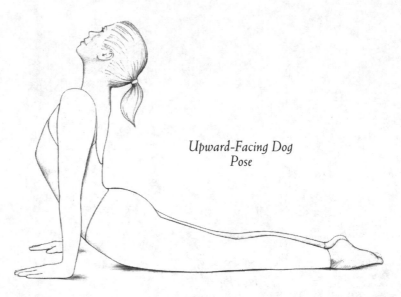

Upward-Facing Dog Pose

11. Exhale; push with your hands and bend at your hips to lift your pelvis upward and back into the Downward-Facing Dog Pose (*Adho Mukha Shvanasana*). (Here's another good spot for more breathing.)

12. Inhale. Lunge, bringing the same foot between your hands as before (in this case, the left), going back into the Monkey Pose (*Banarasana*). Another way to get here is to bring both knees to the floor (you'll be on hands and knees), and from this position step one leg forward into the lunge.

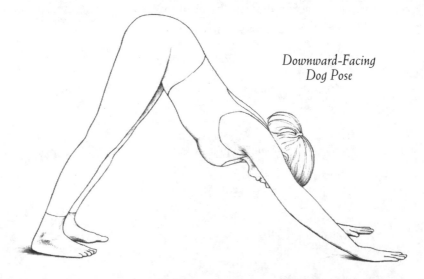

Downward-Facing Dog Pose

13. Exhale. Keeping your hands on the floor, push off from your back toes and your front foot and step your feet close together, side by side. End up folded over, with the top of your head aiming toward the floor, revisiting the Standing Forward Pose (*Uttanasana*). Bend your knees if you need to. (Hold and breathe.)

14. Inhale to hinge all the way up to standing, keeping your arms up and your head between them.

15. Exhale, your arms down to the sides.

Repeat with the left foot stepping back into a lunge. Perform the sequence two to four or more times.

MOVEMENT RESEARCH

Giving corrections in yoga class is tricky business. I've been tugged, pulled on, poked, nearly knocked over, and still did not "get" the teacher's suggestion. In my classes I try to look beyond what is obvious, like the knee not being straight or the collapsed back, and attempt to focus on the student's reasons for performing a pose in a certain way. I realized that I need to see the person, not the pose. To me, the pose is just a format for bringing things out about a person, things you wouldn't notice right away if you were lightly conversing with that individual at a cocktail party. In posture practice nothing is hidden because your body expresses your soul and its struggles at every life turn.

Assisting people in their practice becomes a question of meeting them in their comfort so they will be happy to consider a suggestion that comes out of close and reverent observation of their work in the pose.

I am fascinated by how the different postures reveal our very human complexity and by how yoga's model of our place in the cosmos is a very practical one. This is how the movement research aspect of my work came about. Initially, I observed these distinct stages in a student's progress where intervention on my part was useful:

1. Someone doesn't clearly know what to do or how to do it.

2. Someone is unaware of what her body is actually doing. For example, a person might have limited awareness of where she is tense or how she is breathing.

3. Someone is unable to find alternative ways of doing what needs to be done to improve, even though she recognizes what she was doing is not working.

So I began looking at what my students and clients were doing and analyzing what information or awareness was missing. Then I designed simple movement patterns or exercises to draw awareness to that particular element of practice, whether it had to do with better use of feet in balancing, or reducing anxiety through breath awareness, or rotating the arm fully in the shoulder joint. I called this remedial movement practice.

Remedial Movement

Remedial movement gives you insight into how your body moves and how you are moving your body. It does this by giving you the opportunity to tease out and focus on a universal principle that feeds into perfecting complex poses or posture sequences. The process could be likened to a musician's practice of the scales or her refining techniques that help her to play a particularly difficult passage. Any aspect of yoga practice that stumps you can become the topic. We might work with movements that take the hips through their range of motion, or move in ways that give a sense of how the two bones in the lower legs support balance in relation to the arches of the feet. Sometimes I teach an entire class of remedial movement by introducing each pattern like an ingredient in a recipe for an advanced yoga pose. Then near the end of class we bring our understanding of the various pieces together into the posture.

There are probably a million possible remedial movement practices. One practice may help someone with bunions understand how to better align her legs and knees. Another may remind us of ancient actions that are already part of our basic physiology, actions we can call upon to help organize and streamline our efforts. In this exercise, we will simply move in ways that recall some of these ancient action patterns. I like to think of this as a nervous system tune-up inspired by the work of Bonnie Bainbridge Cohen. We'll focus on four patterns that are hardwired into our nervous system. They provide important support for most moving and held postures. Calling forth these universal movement patterns in yoga practice is like jumping from black and white to color in *The Wizard of Oz*. You'll move in a particular way to search for a hook-up into the pattern. When you tap in during practice, your nervous system recalls the ancient actions on which the postures are based. The experience of these actions takes you deeper into connection with all lifeforms. This may start to sound like New Age dribble, but it is really what happens when you have a direct experience of the power of the forms and underlying patterns of yoga practice. Activate these patterns on a regular basis and your everyday actions will be all the more graceful and efficient. This is valuable to athletes and dancers, but of particular importance to us mere mortals as our bodies age.

We will work from the most complex pattern to the simplest. There are four parts to the practice—diagonal connections, same side coordination, upper-lower activation, and spinal focus—each activating a different pattern. For this one, it is best to be on a surface you can slide over, like a hardwood floor. Focus on the feeling of connection throughout the body rather than the shape your body makes as you practice.

DIAGONAL CONNECTIONS

Rest on your back with your arms wide overhead and your legs spread. Visualize and feel the shape of a big X from opposite hands to feet. As you move, focus on the diagonal lines of energy through your body. Exhale and move your right hand and your left foot off the floor toward each other. (Don't worry, they don't have to touch.) Inhale; move them back to the starting position. Now repeat with the opposite hand and foot. Exhale; move the left hand and the right foot toward each other. Inhale; move them back to the starting position. Alternate many times. If interested, try this on your belly!

Next, move the right elbow to the left knee and back. Then move the left elbow to the right knee and back. Explore these mid-limb diagonal opposites. Finally, move the right shoulder toward the left hip. They can just aim in the direction; simply feel them activate and try to come together, then apart. Repeat with the left shoulder and right hip. Rest for a moment.

SAME SIDE COORDINATION

Begin flat on the floor on your back. Visualize a line running from your head to your tailbone, splitting your body into right and left sides. Feel each side independent of the other. Now bend at the side, remaining flat on the floor, by bringing the right hip and right shoulder toward each another. Then unbend that side and stretch back up to the big X. Repeat several times. Then bend at the side, remaining flat, by bringing the left hip and left shoulder toward one another. Unbend the side and stretch back up to the starting position. Repeat several times. Now repeat the side bend but with the right elbow coming to meet the right knee. Then unbend as before. It is not important how close they get. Don't lift off the floor to twist, but instead, slide on the floor. Repeat with the left elbow and knee leading the side bend. Now try it on each side with your hand and your foot leading. Remember to remain as flat on the floor as possible. Alternate side to side. Rest a moment.

UPPER-LOWER ACTIVATION

Lying on your back, imagine a line at your waist separating the top of your body from the bottom. Draw your legs off the floor by bending your knees and folding your legs up over your torso. As you exhale, curl your tailbone under and lift your pelvis and legs off the floor. Inhale to lower. Place your arms overhead on the floor. Exhale to curl your upper spine forward, bringing your head and upper torso slightly off the floor. Reach your arms forward. Inhale to lower. Repeat each several times. Exhale to lift, inhale to lower. Now alternate. Lift your upper body and lower it; then lift your lower body and lower it. In a similar way as above, you can lead with the elbows and knees or with the hands and feet, splitting your body at the waist. Repeat as much as you like (it's kind of fun!). Rest a moment.

SPINAL FOCUS

Sit on the floor with your knees bent and the soles of your feet placed on the floor slightly away from your torso. If this isn't comfortable, sit on a chair instead. Visualize and feel your entire spine. Focus in its ends—the top of your head and the tip of your tailbone. Inhale and lengthen from head to tailbone. Lift your arms overhead if this helps you to feel long. Exhale and curl your spine into a C shape. You can bring your arms forward to your knees if you like. Then inhale again to elongate, coming back up to a vertical extended position with your arms overhead or relaxed at your sides. Continue this way, focusing on your spine. Once you've tuned in to your spine, play around with spinal movement. Rest.

movement patterns life strategies

The developmental patterns touched on in this moving practice are just the tip of the iceberg of what you can discover about yourself by including movement exploration in your practice. Yielding, pushing, reaching, grasping, and pulling actions, which are all a part of our development, have been left out of the discussion of this exercise. As we grow, we investigate our world and express our needs. To do so, we form increasingly complex behavioral patterns based on rudimentary actions such as these. We learn what works and what doesn't in getting our needs and desires met. We carry these patterns into our lives as life strategies. They are the behavioral superhighways we develop for ourselves. We become yielding or pushy, soft-spined or rigid. Our life strategy patterns are available to us in the static postures (*asanas*) as well. There they exist as distilled actions ripe with information about us. Yoga offers us a way to examine our humanness—not to fix it, but to embrace it fully and in so doing to gain freedom.

After these exercises, you may want to move about freely to see what effects they have had. You can repeat the exercises standing, or you can improvise a movement, extending the feeling of the patterns you have just explored.

As I worked with people on remedial movement, an interesting thing began to happen. As individuals tried out new possibilities for using their bodies in yoga practice, I noticed emotions were often involved. Rather than brushing them aside, my clients and I began to explore the relationship these emotions had with what the body was doing. We discovered through our moving practice that these experiences were rich with meaning, as if our souls were speaking through the movement, giving guidance for us in what mattered most in our lives. The last piece came when we took these lessons back into the postures and posture sequences. They gave us strength and courage, as well as compassion, softness, and acceptance. Through this process we gained insight into how these qualities were taken away from us or squelched in the first place. I call the work that evolved out of remedial movements concept exploration. In this work we embody metaphysical metaphors.

Concept Exploration

Movement research gives us a chance to work outside the box in order to deepen our understanding of ourselves in relation to yoga's practices and principles and in relation to the world in general. Concept exploration gives us the chance to investigate topics that come up as we practice. It helps us tune in to the very specific and personal ways we use our body and what they mean to us. There are usually themes that recur if we stay with our practice long enough. In part 3, "Soul Yoga," we'll delve more deeply into free exploration. At this point, however, we focus on exploring principles or concepts that make themselves apparent in practice, such as how we feel when we accept the weight and volume of the body, what taking a stand feels like, and how the breath can guide us in knowing when and how to exert ourselves and when and how to return to ourselves for recuperation. Such insights guide us through yoga practice and are transferable to all aspects of our lives. We can apply them to the support needed in the Downward-Facing Dog Pose, to carrying groceries up three flights of stairs, or to tapping into the mental toughness required to run a marathon. Concept exploration gives us insight into our beliefs and unconscious wisdom—those things our cells remember, but our minds may have forgotten.

A CONCEPT EXPLORATION PRACTICE

Inhale and follow the natural feeling of expansion. Allow it to radiate out through your body. Exhale and notice the feeling of condensing in the chest. Allow this feeling to include the entire body. Inhale and allow the natural impulse to extend out into space. Let your body reach out in whatever way and however much it wants to. Exhale and allow your body to soften and retreat back to its center. Move out through the space around your body as you inhale. Return back into yourself as you exhale. Explore different ways of going out and coming back. What does it feel like to reach into the space around your body? Which feels familiar? Is one better, easier? What emotional response does this elicit? Is there resistance? If so, how do you experience it?

Do you see how this is simply another way to study yourself? This particular moving yoga practice develops self-awareness and self-confidence as we learn to acknowledge our boundaries, support our reach, and recognize our need to return. What are you interested in learning about yourself? How might you inquire about yourself through movement?

Moving practice offers us a way to practice yoga that is comfortable and malleable. If you've got an "exercise is boring torture" program running in your head, moving practice can help you return to a "moving feels great and is interesting" mind-set. This helps you continue to practice over time.

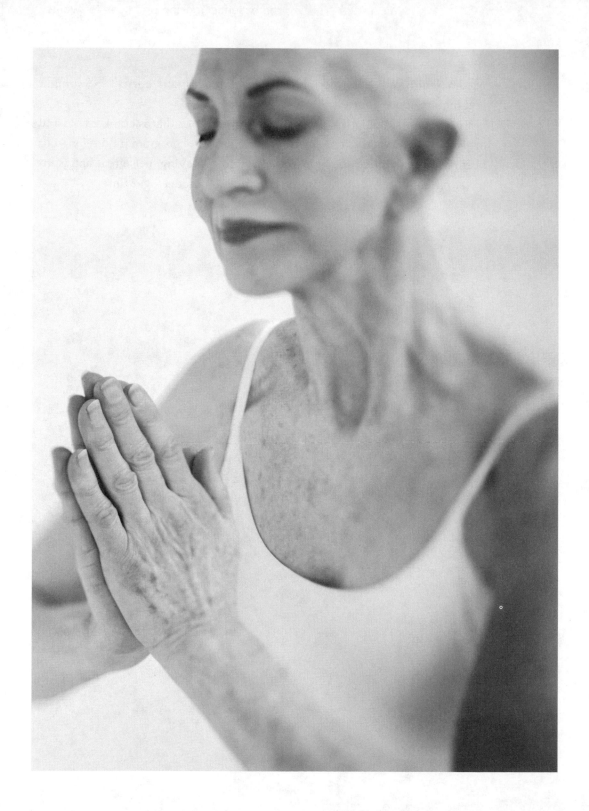

chapter 7

the essential breathing practices

The force that through the green fuse drives the flower
Drives my green age . . .
—Dylan Thomas

All worldly activities are going on only because of the knowledge "I am" to-
gether with that motive force which is the life force, the vital breath. And that is
not something apart from you: you are that only.
—Sri Nisargadatta Maharaj

Once you make posture practice a part of your life, you'll have more long-term energy, more pizzazz, less fizzle. If you practice with attention to your breathing, you'll form a helpful habit that supports your actions throughout the day. You may notice how easily you can pick up a bag of groceries while smoothly exhaling, or that you deeply inhale as you reach up for something on a high shelf. The yoga breathing practices called *pranayama* focus directly on the energy that is the source of life. One definition of *prana* I like is "energy saturated with consciousness." Without it, there is no life or awareness of being alive.

vital breath: the energetic flow of life

Pranayama practices focus directly on vitality. In Sanskrit, words often have more than one meaning. In the compound word *pranayama*, *yama* means con-

on prana

The flow of *prana* drives the mind and produces thoughts. The word *prana* combines two words, *pra* (first unit) and *na* (energy). Everything we can perceive and know is made possible by *prana*. The life of the body is also sustained by *prana*, which is found in the food we eat, in sunlight, and more subtly in the air we breathe. *Prana* is not the chemical nutrients, or the air itself, but the subtle vital energy within them.

Ancient yogic texts such as the Upanishads describe our embodiment in terms of layers of density. The innermost layers consist of mental faculties. They are enclosed in the energetic or *pranic* layer, which in turn is encased in the more dense, physical layer. This model depicts the *pranic* layer, which relates to the breath, as the vital link between mind and body. When your mind is active, it affects your body by modifying the flow of *prana*. Your body's positions and actions also affect this flow, which in turn influences your mind. In *The Science of Breath*, Swami Rama remarks, "Advanced yogis observe that the breath is like a thermometer which registers the conditions of the mind and the influence of the external environment on the body, and those who have studied breath behavior also know their mental and physical behavior." The breath is the most crucial vehicle for *prana* in our bodies. When we work with the breath, we work directly with our own life energy and indirectly with our mental and physical faculties.

trol, so the practices can be a way to harness natural vitality. Through them we are better able to control the mind and emotions and thereby the habits and tendencies that may create havoc in our lives.

When the second word in *pranayama* is taken to be *ayama*, the import changes. *Ayama* means expansion or manifestation. Here *pranayama* means expansion of the life force and promotion of enduring health and longevity. *Pranayama* practices expand and extend the flow of *prana* and bring it under control.

The first step in *pranayama* practice is to become aware of the rate and rhythm of your breath. Becoming sensitive to the motion of breathing and studying the interplay between its automatic movement and our ability to consciously direct it is the starting point of *pranayama* practice. This sensitive awareness is also the entrance into the subtle aspects of our vitality.

PREPARING FOR *PRANAYAMA* PRACTICE

Spending even a moment preparing for an activity gives the mind a chance to transition and focus. Traditionally, one prepares for *pranayama* by washing, if not the entire body, at least the face and hands, and emptying the bladder and bowels if necessary. Most important, the stomach should be empty. The environment for practice should be clean, airy, and quiet.

the diaphragm muscle

The diaphragm separates the torso into two parts. Above it are the heart and lungs; below it are the abdominal organs, such as the stomach, liver, gall bladder, pancreas, and spleen. The diaphragm is made up of a central disc-like tendon with muscles around it that attach to the lower ribs and down the front of the spine. The diaphragm domes up into the chest cavity in its resting state and flattens toward the abdominal cavity when it contracts. This motion is the main action responsible for breathing. As the diaphragm contracts and lowers, a vacuum is created in the chest that draws air into the lungs. As this contraction releases, air is expelled from the lungs. The motion of the diaphragm is automatic. We do not need to think consciously about breathing in order to do it, but we can bring our breath under conscious control, as in speaking and singing.

The best time to practice is before sunrise and after sunset, but finding time before meals may be more practical. If you can find a way to place your practice into your life so that you can do it at the same time of day each time you practice, a positive habit will develop and *pranayama* will easily become a part of your life. Breathe through the nose and approach each practice with ease and kindness toward yourself.

PRANAYAMA PRACTICE

You can do your *pranayama* practice by itself, during the same session as your posture practice, or even in combination with postures. At the end of this chapter, under "*Pranayama* in the Yoga Poses," I give suggestions for trying some of the breathing practices as you perform poses. I squeeze my *pranayama* practice in right after I get dressed. I hide out in the bedroom (my kids think I'm a slow dresser) and do ten minutes of practice before breakfast.

OPTIMAL DIAPHRAGMATIC BREATHING

As the baseline practice, this one increases awareness of how you breathe and improves your ability to breathe naturally and efficiently. The most important thing is to allow your diaphragm to lead in the dance of breathing. Other motions of the chest and abdomen follow in concert with the diaphragm in normal breathing. Optimal breathing requires that the breath travel smoothly and quietly through the nose.

Lie on your back with your feet as wide as your hips or farther apart and your arms eight to ten inches from the sides of your body, palms up. With your eyes closed, place your hands on the soft area of your upper abdomen, below your breastbone and above your waist. Inhale and exhale slowly through your nose, allowing your breath to be smooth, deep, and even. Notice any times when your breath stops or jerks, or when it accelerates or decelerates. See if you can allow the breath motion to become smooth so that your breath cycles as evenly as possible. Do not strain to eliminate pauses. Practice this for three to five minutes. Then stand up and breathe in the same smooth, deep, even way. Take a minimum of six breaths standing.

If this way of breathing is unfamiliar or difficult, make this your *pranayama* practice for at least two months before going on to the other practices in this section. It will be worth it. Deep, even diaphragmatic breathing strengthens the nervous system and helps normalize blood pressure. It's the cornerstone of physical health and mental balance. Regular practice of such a seemingly simple exercise as this increases your lung capacity, vital reserves, and accompanying resistance to environmental pollutants and disease.

HEALING *PRANAYAMA*

This practice involves your imagination. As you inhale through your nostrils, visualize your breath traveling down a central channel to your navel area. This may engender an embryonic quality. You may remember a womb-like connection to sustenance or a sense of personal presence and power. On the exhalation, visualize the *prana* as golden light evenly radiating outward from your navel center to all of your limbs. Include your head and tailbone as limbs. A starburst or blossoming flower can be useful images for sensing evenness. Envision the *prana* delivering vitality to each and every cell.

This *pranayama* is particularly restorative. Use it when you're not well enough to practice postures. Use it on particularly challenging days. Visualizing the vital breath as it radiates *prana* outward from your navel center not only affects the subtle level of pranic flow but permeates all levels of your being. It will bolster the will in healing. Practice for four or more minutes.

2-TO-1 RATIOED BREATHING

There are many yogic patterns of breathing that alter the four aspects of the breath: inhalation, holding the breath in, exhalation, and holding the breath out. Practices that involve breath retention require the guidance of an experienced teacher. But one such practice that does not involve holding the breath, yet gives a sense of the profound effect of altering the even natural breath rhythm, is 2-to-1 Ratioed Breathing. It is done by exhaling for twice the amount of time it takes to inhale. This 2-to-1 Ratioed Breathing strengthens the diaphragm and quiets the nervous system.

Lie supine or sit in a chair. Prepare by allowing your breath to flow evenly with the inhalation taking about the same amount of time as the exhalation. You may wish to count the amount of time it takes for both the inhalation and exhalation. A count of six or eight is usually what an entire breath cycle takes, with three or four counts marking the length of the exhalation and the inhalation.

ratioed breathing

Even optimal diaphragmatic breathing helps to regulate the functioning of the autonomic nervous system. The autonomic nervous system is one aspect of the nervous system that directs our vital functions automatically, without our conscious intervention. The autonomic nervous system divides into the sympathetic and parasympathetic nervous systems. The *sympathetic nervous system* activates the body, enabling it to meet the demands of physical exertion. The *parasympathetic nervous system* prepares the body for digestion, relaxation, and sleep. The thoughts we think and the activities we find ourselves engaged in call into service one or the other of these two systems. Thus not only our actions but our thoughts affect our vital functions.

During the two phases of the breath cycle, each branch of the autonomic nervous system is alternately stimulated. During inhalation, the sympathetic system is emphasized, and during exhalation, the parasympathetic system is stimulated. Changing the ratio of inhalation to exhalation alters the emphasis given to sympathetic and parasympathetic activities during each breath cycle. The 2-to-1 Ratioed Breathing supports relaxation by extending the period of time for parasympathetic activity within each breath.

Slightly shortening your inhalation will make doubling the exhalation easier. Without changing the duration of your entire breath cycle, lengthen the exhalation. If you were inhaling for three counts and exhaling for three counts, now inhale for two and exhale for four. This is a way to achieve a 2-to-1 proportion without strain. Once you're comfortable with this, extend the duration of the inhalation and the exhalation to 4-to-8, or longer. If, on the other hand, you can't yet create a proportion in which the exhalation takes twice as long as the inhalation, just lengthen the exhalation to any duration that is longer than the inhalation. From there you can gradually work toward doubling the exhalation.

This is a valuable *pranayama* practice in its own right, but is also a useful preparation to meditation, as it quiets the nervous system and mind, availing our sensitivities to more subtle realms of experience. In addition, 2-to-1 Ratioed Breathing can be used during moderate aerobic exercise, such as walking, to more fully expel waste and increase the intake of fresh air.

UJJAYI BREATHING

Ujjayi breathing calms the mind, soothes the nerves, and increases internal awareness while inducing overall relaxation. It also reduces phlegm and helps to clear the nasal passages. *Ujjayi* translates to "up" and "victory" and indicates the conquest of physical and psychological imbalances attributed to the upward-flowing aspect of *prana* known as *uddana*.

To prepare, sit in a stable position so your head, neck, and torso are aligned vertically. You may wish to sit on a firm chair with your feet touching the floor or sit cross-legged on the floor. Breathe slowly and fully, feeling the air in both nostrils.

The unique element of this practice is that the glottis in the throat (located just behind the Adam's apple) is partially closed, so that a soft unvoiced sound emanates. It's like whispering with your mouth shut. In our children's class, we call it "Darth Vader Breathing." One way to find this partial closure of the glottis is to speak in a whisper, then close your mouth and breathe with that same quality of tension in your throat. As you breathe, you'll hear a soft sibilant "sss" as you inhale and an aspirant "hhh" as you exhale. Sense the passage of the breath on the roof of the palate. You can keep the abdominal muscles slightly pulled in as you inhale, as this will slightly expand your chest. This expansion can be included as part of the practice.

Practice seated for three to five minutes. Once you've established a habit of breathing this way, practice *ujjayi* breathing lying down or even while walking. It is also a wonderful addition to non-strenuous postures and dynamic posture practice. *Ujjayi* breathing is completely safe and enormously beneficial for everyone.

ALTERNATE NOSTRIL BREATHING (Nadi Shodhanam)

If you are just breezing through this section, don't skip this one! This practice will, as Sly Stone puts it, "take you higher!" *Nadi Shodhanam*, also called alternate nostril breathing, is a traditional *pranayama* practice with many variations. It is used to purify the *pranic* channels or *nadis*, which number seventy-two thousand, originating near the navel and running throughout the entire body.

Like optimal diaphragmatic breathing, this practice restores a sense of calm and balances the nervous energy of the body. You will find yourself in a state of calm, focused attention after practicing for even a few minutes, so it is very useful in everyday situations such as prior to an important meeting or when thoughts or emotions get the better of you. It's a great practice to clear your head! The practice described below is a safe and simple variation. Five to ten minutes of *Nadi Shodhanam* gives you plenty of benefit. However, you may wish to investigate this practice while walking or while waiting in line at the bank or supermarket.

Nadi Shodhanam is marked by slowly and gently alternating the breath from one nostril to the other. After you have found a stable erect position of the spine and renewed optimal diaphragmatic breathing, determine which nostril is freer by closing one nostril and blowing air out the other nostril alternately. You may find that one nostril is dominant or more open than the other, or that they are about even. The thumb of the right hand is used to close the right nostril, and the ring finger is used to close the left nostril. The other fingers can be folded in.

Begin *Nadi Shodhanam* by exhaling first through the nostril that is freer. If both nostrils are free and the breath between them feels even, simply choose

alternate nostril breathing (*nadi shodhanam*)

The *nadis* can be likened to the meridians of Chinese medicine, as they are subtle passageways of energy and not actual anatomical components. Because the vital energy moves in currents through them, they are sometimes associated with nerve impulses and the balanced activity of the nervous system. *Nadi Shodhanam* focuses on the three central *nadis*—the *ida*, *pingala,* and *sushumna*—which run the length of the spine and terminate in the head. The *ida nadi,* in the left nostril, is activated when the breath moves primarily through the left nostril. When the breath moves primarily through the right nostril, the *pingala nadi* is activated. The *sushumna nadi* is centrally located, terminating at the base of the skull. It is activated when the breath moves freely through both nostrils. Through *Nadi Shodhanam* you can experience a state of serenity known as "joyous mind," during which the flow of breath is balanced evenly between the nostrils.

Other benefits of *Nadi Shodhanam* are felt in subtle ways. One such benefit is becoming more attuned to the subtle energies of your body. Awareness of subtle energy could enable you to sense an imbalance in your body before you actually become physically sick. If you maintain a regular yoga practice, you may be able to correct the situation through yogic techniques and circumvent descending into illness.

one (notice I didn't say "pick"). Once you've exhaled through the free nostril, close it and inhale through the less free nostril. This is one breath cycle. Repeat this twice more. Then begin by exhaling through the more clogged nostril and inhaling through the free one. Repeat this twice more. You have now done three cycles beginning with one nostril and three cycles beginning with the opposite nostril. Continue this pattern of three breaths cycling in one direction and three breaths cycling in the other direction for five to ten minutes. You may notice by the end of the practice that the dominance of the nostrils is different from when you began, perhaps becoming more even.

KAPALABHATI

Kapalabhati literally translated means "the *pranayama* that makes the skull shine." It is a potent cleansing technique and an invigorating energetic practice.

Because this is such a powerful exercise, begin with the minimal number of repetitions. Your stomach must be empty. If you have high blood pressure, have heart disease, or experience dizziness, do not include this exercise in your *pranayama* practice. If you discontinue regular practice, you must start again at the beginning, not with the number of repetitions at which you left off. When you perform *Kapalabhati*, do not intentionally hold your breath—either in or

on *kapalabhati*

Besides clearing the sinuses and air passageways, *Kapalabhati* removes toxins from the body's tissues via the lungs. It emphasizes a quick and strong exhalation, which increases the amount of waste expelled through the lung tissue. As the volume of air passing through the lungs increases, the blood flow through them and throughout the entire body is increased as well. As with any cleansing practice, once waste is removed from an organ of elimination, the body further releases toxins to that organ for removal. This is something like emptying the wastebasket so you can fill it again. Expelling waste through the lungs reduces the burden of elimination on the liver, colon, kidneys, and skin. This practice dramatically strengthens the diaphragm and abdominal wall. Without even one sit-up, regular practice of *Kapalabhati* can strengthen the muscles of the belly wall. The motions of the diaphragm and abdominal muscles stimulate the abdominal and digestive organs, such as the stomach, colon, liver, spleen, and pancreas.

out—because you might pass out. If you experience pain, dizziness, an ache in your side, or you're unable to maintain a steady rhythm, stop! My rule is this: "When in doubt, don't do it!" You can always check out this or any other yoga practice with your doctor.

Prepare by sitting in a stable, erect position. Establish even optimal diaphragmatic breathing. Exhale and sense the movement of the diaphragm. Near the end of the exhalation, contract your abdominal muscles from your pubic bone up to your ribs. Notice that more air is pressed out. Relax and allow the air to enter your lungs without any effort on your part.

This time, exhale quickly and pull your abdominal wall back in one sudden powerful action. Relax and passively allow the air to flow into your lungs. This is one breath cycle of *Kapalabhati*. Repeat this seven to ten times. Because your body usually works harder to inhale than to exhale, this pattern may strike you as odd. Practice making the exhalation forceful and the inhalation relaxed. You will probably take roughly twice as long to inhale as you do to exhale in this practice. Keep the repetitions rhythmic. Also check to see if you are slumping forward or hunching your shoulders up, as these add unnecessary tension and inhibit breathing.

Once you familiarize yourself with the feeling of the practice, begin with seven to ten repetitions done in three sets, with time for the breath to normalize between sets. Add a few repetitions to each set per week until you reach twenty repetitions per set. This would be twenty repetitions for three sets. The benefits come with regular practice. When you come to the maximum number of repetitions recommended here, and you wish to do more or to explore related vigorous practices, seek out the guidance of a teacher with experience in *pranayama*.

Kapalabhati can be practiced in conjunction with certain postures and is useful whenever you want to recharge your batteries. It's great after work before dinner, as it stimulates the digestive fire and gives you energy to cook the meal. Because it cleans the blood and stimulates the cardiovascular system, it is useful when you simply can't exercise, such as when you're on a hectic business trip or you're snowbound with a baby.

VOCALIZATION

While not a *pranayama* practice in the classical sense, vocalizing a syllable or simple word for the duration of an exhalation strengthens the diaphragm and brings it more under conscious control. It also activates parasympathetic activity of the autonomic nervous system (the relaxation side) in the same way described in 2-to-1 Ratioed Breathing by emphasizing the exhalation. Perhaps this aspect of singing and chanting factors into the sense of renewal it brings.

The sacred sound of "Om" (*Aum*), the vibratory representation of the total sound of the universe, is worthy of use. If you prefer, however, other single vowel sounds such as short "a" (ah) or long "u" (oo) will suffice.

Begin by sitting in an erect position; take in a hearty breath. Now sustain the sound you have chosen for the duration of the exhale. Near the end, you'll be able to breathe out just a bit longer than you're able to make a sound. Allow your breath to enter slowly into your body. Any pitch will do. Explore different notes, keeping your attention on feeling your breath. Do this with friends to make a most intriguing soundscape.

PRANAYAMA IN THE YOGA POSES

Even diaphragmatic breathing is a necessary starting point in properly performing yoga poses (*asanas*) and dynamic sequences (*vinyasa krama*). It's the groundwork for yoga practice. Once well established, altering the breath ratio or adding *Ujjayi* breathing intensifies concentration and benefit. Although best learned in person with an experienced teacher, you may want to explore adding a specific *pranayama* to part of your posture practice. For example, in the seated forward bend (*Paschimottanasana*), extend the exhalation. Breathe in for four counts and exhale for eight. This breathing pattern helps slow the pulse to support relaxation in this pose.

If you struggle with keeping your breath even, you may want to add *Ujjayi* breathing to your posture practice. It gives audible feedback to the rate and rhythm of your breath while soothing the nerves. To try this, lie prone, hands next to your chest, for the Cobra Pose. Lift your head, upper torso, and back while maintaining a long, controlled *Ujjayi* inhalation. Stay up there, making the ocean-sounding breath for one exhalation and one more inhalation. Then slowly return to the floor as you exhale. Did you maintain the *Ujjayi* breath sound? Were you better able to observe the steadiness of your breath by hearing it? Was it easy or difficult? Explore these two breathing options with your posture practice. Seek expert guidance for more advanced and interesting combinations.

YOUR OWN *PRANAYAMA* PRACTICE

It's best to choose one or two practices to do regularly, daily if possible. Give yourself time to learn all these methods, and then include them as options to your basic practice. A few minutes of optimal diaphragmatic breathing, followed by a few minutes of healing *pranayama* or *Ujjayi* breathing, would be a good basis for a beginning *pranayama* practice. Throughout the course of the week, you could select one of the other practices, adding a different one each day to your basic practice. Another possibility is to do *Kapalabhati*, followed by *Nadi Shodanam*, and then vocalization. This sequence is a wonderful preparation for meditation. Or you could begin with optimal diaphragmatic breathing, transition into *Ujjayi* breathing, and finish with 2-to-1 Ratioed Breathing to ensure a sound night's sleep. Once you make these practices your own, study their effects on your energy and state of mind. You'll be the expert on how *pranayama* supports your health, clarity, respite, and vigor over the course of your life.

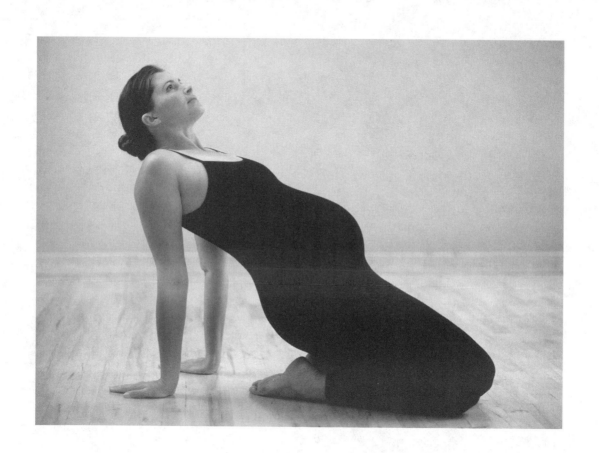

chapter 8

restoring balanced health:
yoga practices for
special times and needs

Sickness is Nature's tap on the shoulder, Her reminder to you that you have strayed from the path.

—Dr. Robert Svoboda

Working experientially with the breath, and watching things shift within and around you, is quite different from the sort of spiritual pursuit that involves abstract discussions by theologians. It's also more relevant to that process of reorganization we call healing.

—Dr. Rudolf Ballentine

When we use yoga methods for specific problems, we establish the conditions for balanced health. Natural healing relies on our innate ability to seek equilibrium. Western health care offers miraculous innovations in relief of symptoms. It can get us out of sticky situations brought on by the little inequities we engage in that chip away at our health. However, relying on Western health care can be like having a big brother on the playground; we can become cavalier in our ways because we think we are protected. The convenience and reassurance of the silver bullet allow us to ignore harmful patterns of behavior that throw us out of balance in the first place.

We are complex, resilient beings living in a world of constant change. The therapeutic application of yoga considers a multitude of interactive factors in our health: thought patterns, disposition, conditioned responses to biological urges, constitution, heredity, life strategies, personal beliefs and upbringing, cultural myths and taboos, diet, education, career, and relationships. Yoga practice involves every part of us. I am always amused and a bit curious when yoga is marketed as only an exercise regimen. How strange! If you work out, you know that any physical training involves all of you—emotional motivation, will, perseverance, mental concentration. The physical *is* metaphysical. There is no true separation. Yoga's teachings acknowledge the importance of awareness in physical experience in transforming our lives.

Perhaps we're frightened to look inside ourselves. Yoga is very helpful here. It teaches us to look with dispassion, not with judgment left over from some earlier experience. In fact, yoga's method of self-transformation is twofold. First, it helps us to examine the many factors in our lives that lead to imbalanced health. With persistence and dispassion, we tease apart the influences and behaviors at the root of our dilemma. This self-study and discrimination empower us to extricate ourselves from unhealthy habits and associations. Second, yoga offers an assortment of beneficial mental, emotional, and physical practices—such as meditation, breath, posture, and movement practice—that support change at many levels that promote balanced health.

Through yoga we cultivate compassion for ourselves and for others because we observe that our personality is a great big habit conditioned by the strategies and beliefs we have adopted up to this point. Yoga is not at all about a guilt trip. It is not about blame or holding on. Yoga helps us to dismantle damaging self-judgmental conditioning. If we're brave enough to sort through the habits we cling to, we begin to see that they are in fact the chains that keep us fettered to our misery. Therapeutic yoga practice puts the tools for freedom in our very own inner-guided hands.

I have drawn on Ayurvedic principles. *Ayurveda* is a Sanskrit word that means "knowledge of life" and is an ancient system of health care that focuses on longevity and immunity. Its roots are intermingled with yoga, dating back three thousand to five thousand years. Like yoga, Ayurveda considers the uniqueness of each person in her totality—mind, body, and soul—in relation to the intricate workings of nature.

These recommendations are meant to gently guide your exploration. Choose a variation of any suggested practice that suits you best right now. Pay attention to how each practice affects you. Your very personal path to regaining balance requires that you monitor the effects with sensitivity and awareness. Are these practices exactly right for you just now? If not, which ones aren't? Ask yourself what is needed and how to modify these suggestions. Your ability to know will improve as you practice.

Get assistance from an experienced yoga therapist for help in tailoring practices to your needs. Of course, these suggestions are not intended as a substitute for professional medical treatment; but with your health care provider's approval, they can complement Western medical practices. The following issue-related practice routines can be used as the basis of your regular practice.

Finally, these suggestions will only help you if you do them! *Abhyasa, abhyasa, abhyasa!* (Practice, practice, practice!) Yoga practice is a powerful tool in establishing and maintaining balanced health, but it will take you only so far if you lose sight of healthful lifestyle choices. The Seven Treasures of Balanced Health in chapter 12 provides guidance in this area.

conditions central to being female

Open channels of expression are a sign of empowered health.

A healthy woman cultivates situations that support her unique expression of being in the world. She feels free to express herself through the choices she makes. She invests in supportive relationships and engages in meaningful activities that in turn nourish her. Being female in our culture is complicated by the commerce-driven bombardment of messages we receive daily about who we are, how we should look and be, and what should be important to us.

Yoga is a way to understand how our body's state of health reflects what we are struggling with in our lives.

Even though the suggestions below may seem mechanical at first, get into them. Once into the experience of practice, you will have placed yourself in a numinous space of self-discovery. Allow yourself to take action from these places. Don't approach this as a job, but as a love affair with your Self. I am a very hands-off teacher and therapist. I believe my job is to guide but not to direct. Some people don't like my classes. They want to be told what to do every moment, even how many times to breathe in each pose. I want them to reconnect immediately with inner sensing and develop skill in negotiating the terrain of their body and mind. Yoga is very empowering if you take the reins. Part of developing skill involves trying things out. Sometimes they don't work, so you adjust and go on. Do that here. Grab the reins.

MENSTRUAL ISSUES

The regularity and ease of your menstrual cycle is an indicator of your overall health. In Ayurveda, *prajnaparadha* ("crimes against wisdom") refers to the little injustices we all do to ourselves that we know we shouldn't do. We eat too much before bed; work late and skip exercise; choose coffee, diet soda, and chips over regular meals too often. It may not be until a few days before menstruation begins that we notice the effects of these little wrongs, but like the devoted mother, nature has been keeping track. Women have the blessing of monthly purification. When we stray, we pay . . . by the month.

A host of causative factors may contribute to menstrual irregularities, cramps, and symptoms of premenstrual syndrome (PMS). A consistent basic yoga practice has a powerful effect. Practice Hatha Yoga on the days when you're not menstruating to promote menstrual regularity. Poor lifestyle choices negate much of this effort so combine your practice with attention to the Seven Treasures outlined in chapter 12. Check with a doctor first to find out if your symptoms are a sign of more serious illness.

The practices suggested below harmonize hormonal production through subtle manipulation of glands and direct potent energy in specific patterns through the *nadis* (energy channels). Their focus is to strengthen the whole reproductive system.

To focus practice on menstrual regularity and reproductive health, make these postures a part of your regular practice during the days of the month when you're not menstruating.

1. Solar Energizer (*Agni Sara*)

2. Sun Salutation (*Surya Namaskara*), extending the length of time in Downward-Facing Dog Pose (*Adho Mukha Shvanasana*) and Standing Forward Fold Pose (*Uttanasana*)

3. Cobra Pose (*Bhujangasana*)

4. Locust Pose (*Shalabhasana*) or Half Locust Pose (*Ardha Shalabhasana*)

5. Bow Pose (*Dhanurasana*) or Half Bow Pose (*Ardha Dhanurasana*)

6. Symbol of Yoga Pose (*Yoga Mudrasana*) (pose not pictured, see page 106)

7. Posterior Stretch Pose (*Paschimottanasana*)

8. Inverted Action Pose (*Viparita Karani*) or Shoulder Stand Pose (*Sarvangasana*) or Supported Inversion Poses, Version 2 (Feet up Wall) or Version 3 (The Perfect Wedge)

9. Plow Pose (*Halasana*)

10. Half Fish Pose (*Ardha Matsyasana*)

11. Basic Relaxation Pose (*Shavasana*) or Supported Relaxation Pose with Vocalization *Pranayama*

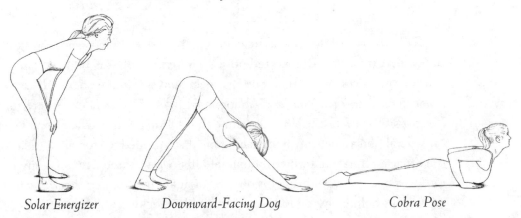

Solar Energizer   *Downward-Facing Dog*   *Cobra Pose*

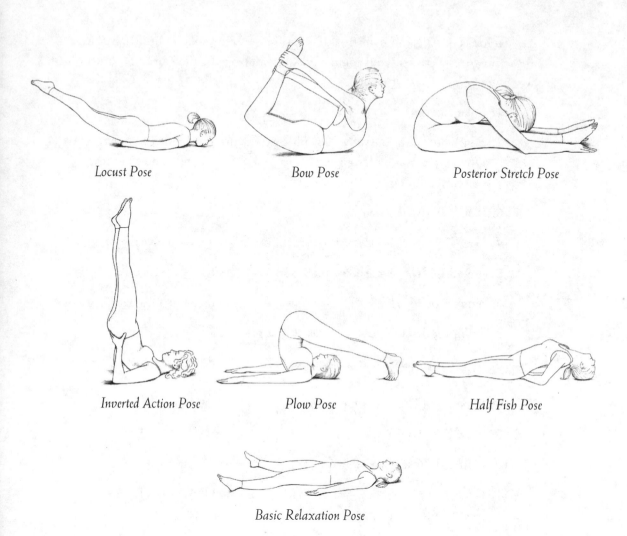

Locust Pose

Bow Pose

Posterior Stretch Pose

Inverted Action Pose

Plow Pose

Half Fish Pose

Basic Relaxation Pose

The downward flow of subtle energy in the body, called *apana prana*, initiates menstruation. All inverted poses, where the pelvis is higher than the heart, or practices whose action brings energy upward in the body, such as the Solar Energizer (*Agni Sara*) and Abdominal Lifts (*Uddiyana Bandha*), interrupt and possibly negate this flow. I've done this. During a time when I practiced for several hours a day, my body taught me that I needed to stop all inversions, the Solar Energizer, and the Abdominal Lifts two to three days *before* my period was due or I wouldn't get it on time or at all. If I stopped these practices a few days before, my period would come like clockwork. I was used to running long distances, dancing for hours, working two shifts, and other exhausting exertions, all with my period right as rain. But those yoga practices stopped it.

Most yoga traditions widely agree it is best not to do these types of practices during the days of your heaviest flow, which are usually the first three days. More conservative schools teach that it's best to skip Hatha Yoga practice altogether during your menses. You might actually increase cramping and cause excessive bleeding in some instances. Yoga teaches us to develop sensitivity to our own body's feedback and needs. Your body will tell you what is right for you, depending on your own system. It is often recommended that you use this time for relaxation practice, meditation, and reflection. *Apana prana* is moving energy down and out of your body as a natural process. Why struggle against this?

Having said all that, I realize there are times when a little movement or stretching gives relief for the cramps or heaviness you feel in your lower body and back. The poses below are options that you may already have found your body doing automatically to give relief for discomfort.

For times of menstrual discomfort, select from these poses:

1. Cat Stretch (*Bidalasana*) from Gentle Limbering Side Bar in chapter 3 (pose not pictured; see page 39)

2. Reclined Hero Pose (*Supta Virasana*) or Reclined Half Hero Pose (*Ardha Supta Virasana*) (pose not pictured; see page 107)

3. Child's Pose (*Balasana*)

4. Bound Angle Pose (*Baddha Konasana*)

5. Reclined Bound Angle Pose (*Supta Baddha Konasana*)

6. Head-to-Knee Pose (*Janu Shirshasana*)

7. Posterior Stretch Pose (*Paschimottanasana*)

8. Spread Leg Pose (*Upavishtha Konasana*)

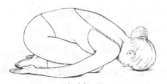
Child's Pose

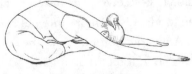
Bound Angle Pose

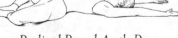
Reclined Bound Angle Pose

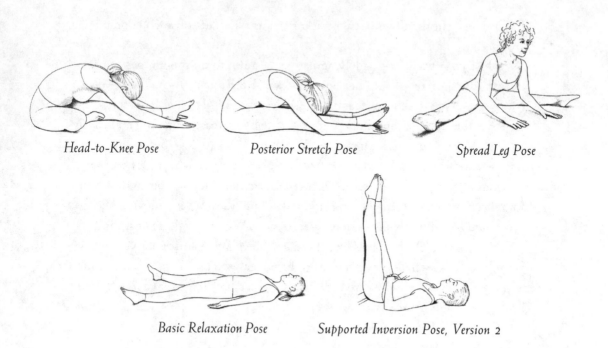

Head-to-Knee Pose   Posterior Stretch Pose   Spread Leg Pose

Basic Relaxation Pose   Supported Inversion Pose, Version 2

9. Basic Relaxation Pose (*Shavasana*)

10. Supported Inversion Pose, Version 1 or Version 2

INABILITY TO BECOME PREGNANT

Infertility is defined by the failure to conceive after a year or more of trying without contraception, or in the case of conception, after three miscarriages. In looking for the source of the problem, we must consider so many variables in both partners and in their relationship that it's a wonder there are so many people in the world! Such is testimony to nature's force compared to our personal designs. In my yoga therapy work with women trying to become pregnant, I've noticed that the label *infertile* is sometimes declared too soon and may be attributed to impatience (demanding that nature instantaneously comply with a decision to conceive). For instance, after coming off the pill, the body requires time to adjust to a more integral hormonal rhythm.

From an Ayurvedic point of view, the conditions necessary for conception in our body are no different than for any other fertile ground. Fertility requires four factors to be functioning and in place:

Season (*rtu*), referring to a regular menstrual cycle

Field (*kshetra*), a healthy womb and associated organs

Seed (*bija*), your ovum and his sperm

Juice (*rasa*), which refers to the purity and health of your blood, balance of hormones, and other ingredients that will nourish your "seedling" as it grows within

I have heard overworked, competitively thin women who are ambivalent about what motherhood will do to their lives and their figures complain about infertility. Dietary extremes, caffeine, and excessive exercise have dried out their juice (*rasa*) to the point of disrupting their cycle (*rtu*). An imbalance in one fertility factor can contribute to the demise of another.

Attention to the Seven Treasures of Balanced Health (detailed in chapter 12) is not trifling in the case of infertility. Also check with your doctor. A different angle is to search for emotional conflicts that may be dictating your body's state of being. What messages is your partner giving you subliminally or otherwise about parenting and his commitment to you? Is there anything from childhood that could have an influence on your becoming a mother?

Till your garden to prepare for pregnancy by making these practices part of your regular routine:

1. Solar Energizer (*Agni Sara*) with focus on Root Lock (*Mula Bandha*)

2. Supported Inversion Poses, Version 2 (Feet up Wall) or Version 3 (The Perfect Wedge) or Shoulder Stand Pose (*Sarvangasana*) or Inverted Action Pose (*Viparita Karani*)

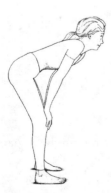
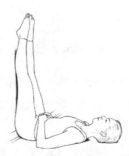
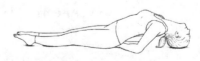

Solar Energizer   *Supported Inversion Pose, Version 2*   *Half Fish Pose*

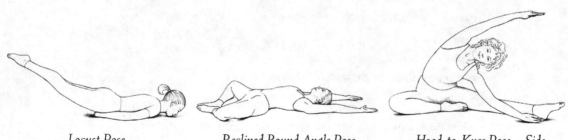

Locust Pose   Reclined Bound Angle Pose   Head-to-Knee Pose—Side

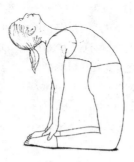

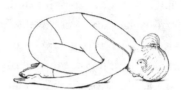

Camel Pose   Child's Pose

3. Half Fish Pose (*Ardha Matsyasana*). Use Plow Pose (*Halasana*) as transition from Shoulder Stand.

4. Locust Pose (*Shalabhasana*)

5. Reclined Bound Angle Pose (*Supta Baddha Konasana*)

6. Head-to-Knee Pose (*Janu Shirshasana*): Forward and Side

7. Camel Pose (*Ushtrasana*) or Half Camel Pose (*Ardha Ushtrasana*)

8. Child's Pose (*Balasana*)

9. 2-to-1 Ratioed Breathing (not pictured; see page 157)

10. *Ujjayi Pranayama* (not pictured; see page 159)

11. Alternate Nostril Breathing (*Nadi Shodhanam*) (not pictured; see page 159)

12. *Kapalabhati Pranayama* (not pictured; see page 161)

VAGINAL HEALTH

If you were to choose a potted plant at a garden store, you would look for the one with the darkest green leaves, the one that had a luster and slightly oily touch. You'd pick the one that looked bold and perked up with juiciness. This plant would be most resistant to disease. If you looked around and saw a yellowing plant, you'd know it would be the one that parasites would attack because they would have an easy time of it.

The same natural principle applies to us. When we deplete our reserves, dimming our brightness (*tejas*) and compromising our resistance (*ojas*), we make our bodies vulnerable to predators, microscopic or otherwise. Lifestyle stress, such as overwork, lack of sleep, anxiety, and nervous tension, leaves us run down and is often at the root of poor dietary choices. Foods like refined sugar, fat, dairy, and wheat in excess clog the body's natural ability to cleanse. Both depletion and toxicity predispose us toward excessive vaginal discharge, which is a perfect site for infection. Seek professional help if you're having an outbreak. To help prevent one, cut down on refined foods, especially sugar, and fortify your diet with yellow/orange (for cleansing) and green (for nourishing) vegetables. Add an internal cleansing regime.

Some other causes of vaginal discharge are hormonal imbalance, birth control, and emotional factors. A steady practice of Hatha Yoga is purifying, as well as strengthening. Unconscious feelings and beliefs may come to the surface during practice as you develop the capacity to receive this information and transform it. None of the poses act on us at only the physical level. Each one stirs vital energy in a different way.

These postures will have a positive effect on your reproductive system because of their focus on your glands and pelvic organs. There are a lot of backward-bending poses here. Unless you're in excellent condition, don't do them all in one practice session. Select a few today, the others tomorrow.

Practice for Reproductive Support

1. Sun Salutation (*Surya Namaskara*) (pose not pictured; see appendix E)

2. Cat Stretch (*Bidalasana*)—from Gentle Limbering side bar in chapter 3 (pose not pictured; see page 39)

3. Cobra Pose (*Bhujangasana*)

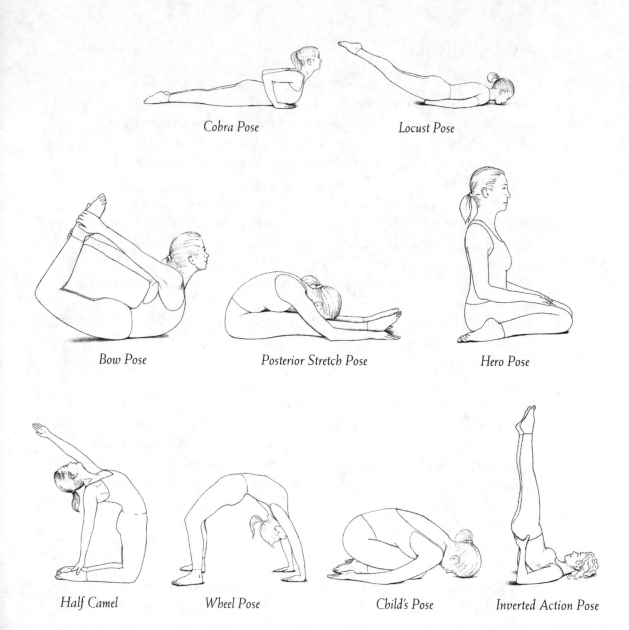

Cobra Pose

Locust Pose

Bow Pose

Posterior Stretch Pose

Hero Pose

Half Camel

Wheel Pose

Child's Pose

Inverted Action Pose

4. Locust Pose (*Shalabhasana*) or Half Locust Pose (*Ardha Shalabhasana*)

5. Bow Pose (*Dhanurasana*) or Half Bow Pose (*Ardha Dhanurasana*)

6. Posterior Stretch Pose (*Paschimottanasana*)

7. Hero Pose (*Virasana*) or Reclined Hero Pose (*Supta Virasana*)

8. Half Camel Pose (*Ardha Ushtrasana*) or Camel Pose (*Ushtrasana*)

9. Wheel Pose (*Chakrasana*)

10. Child's Pose (*Balasana*)

11. Inverted Action Pose (*Viparita Karani*) or Shoulder Stand Pose (*Sarvangasana*) or Supported Inversion Poses, Version 2 (Feet up Wall) or Version 3 (The Perfect Wedge)

PREGNANCY

During the first three months of pregnancy, it is safe to continue with most Hatha Yoga practices. However, double leg lifts, breath retention, intense abdominal contractions, and extreme backward arches with arms overhead are potentially harmful. As the size of the fetus increases, you will benefit most from practices that relieve the discomfort of carrying a baby. As the delivery date approaches, prepare with supported relaxation practices and meditative techniques. Include gentle aerobic activities like swimming or walking in your daily routine. As the uterus becomes heavy, some women experience lower blood pressure and reduced blood flow to the fetus when resting on their back or in shoulder stands. For this reason, it is prudent to relax on your side instead and discontinue shoulder stands after the fourth month. In general, inverted poses will interrupt the natural downward flow of subtle energy (*apana prana*), which is necessary for normal delivery. Cautious experts advise refraining from all inverted poses during pregnancy. This is a time for moderation, quiet, and calm mental clarity in preparation for the big event. The awareness you cultivate now will serve you well during the birthing process.

A Basic Prenatal Practice

1. Root Lock (*Mula Bandha*), yoga's Kegel exercises

2. Supported Revolved Triangle Pose (*Parivritta Trikonasana*)—Make It Easier version

3. Supported Warrior Pose (*Virabhadrasana*)

4. Standing Forward Fold Pose (*Uttanasana*)—Make It Easier version

5. Bound Angle Pose (*Baddha Konasana*)

6. Spread Leg Pose (*Upavishtha Konasana*)

7. Upward-Facing Plank Pose (*Purvottanasana*)

8. Desk Pose (*Dvipada Pitham*)

9. Abdominal Stretch Pose (*Jathara Parivritta*)

10. Flapping Fish Pose (*Matsya Kridasana*)

11. *Yoni Mudra* (see sidebar)

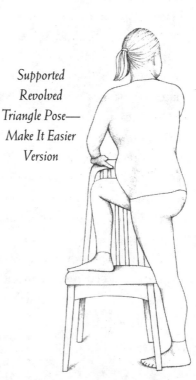

Supported Revolved Triangle Pose— Make It Easier Version

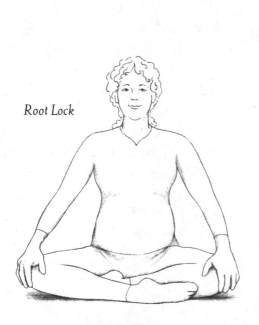

Root Lock

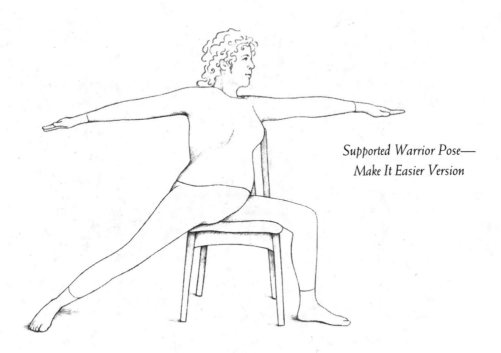

Supported Warrior Pose—
Make It Easier Version

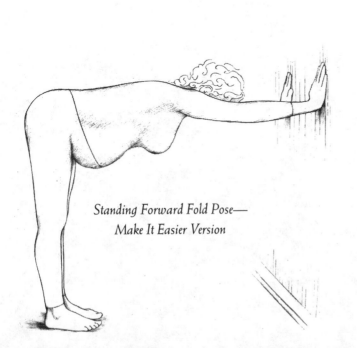

Standing Forward Fold Pose—
Make It Easier Version

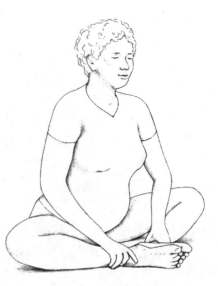

Bound Angle Pose

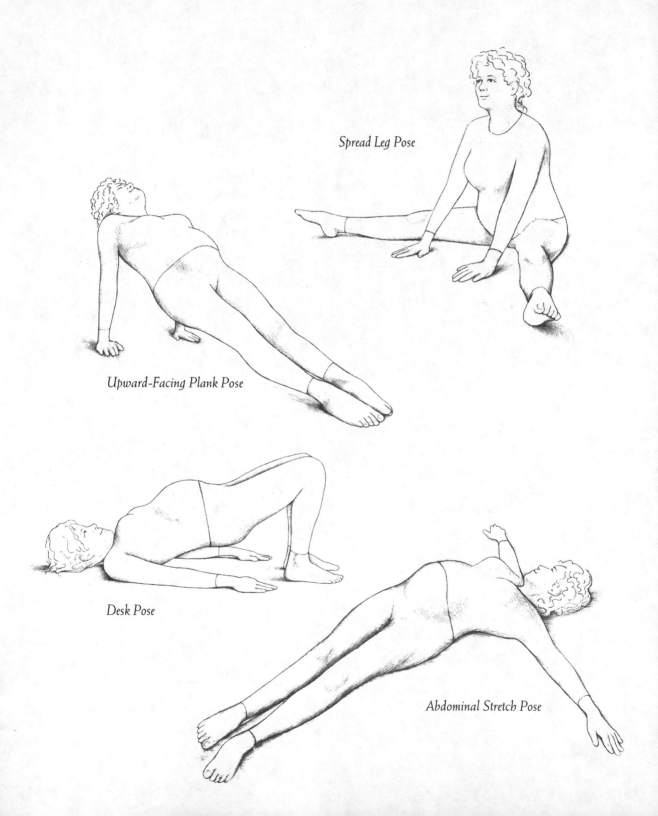

Spread Leg Pose

Upward-Facing Plank Pose

Desk Pose

Abdominal Stretch Pose

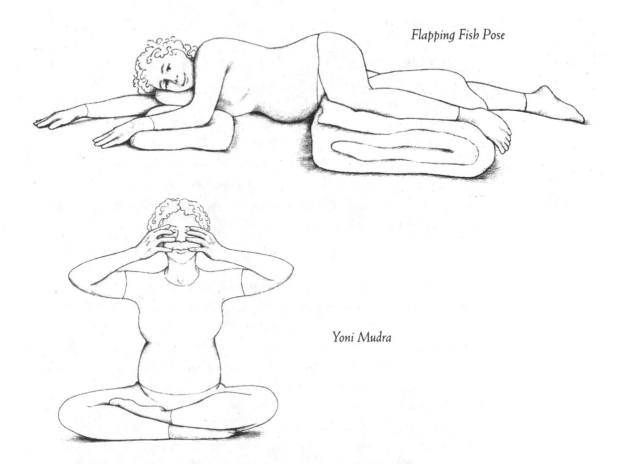

Flapping Fish Pose

Yoni Mudra

yoni mudra (sensory withdrawal practice)

Yoni means "womb" and *mudra* means "seal." This practice closes the gates on the outward-attending senses to allow you to focus on inner sensing. It helps quiet the mind and the nerves, redirecting attention to the inner world. It can provide the peace needed to prepare for the huge life transition of motherhood. If you're already on board, it gives an inner focused breathing space away from the fray.

Sit erect and cover your face with your hands like this: Place your thumbs gently in your ear holes, place your index fingers on your eyebrows, the middle fingers very gently on closed eyelids. Touch the tips of your ring fingers on the outer sides of the nostrils and your small fingers on the corners of your mouth. Remain here with even, long breathing for as long as you like.

MENOPAUSE

> In Celtic cultures, the young maiden was seen as the flower; the
> mother, the fruit; the elder woman, the seed. The seed is the part that
> contains the knowledge and potential of all the other parts within it.
> The role of the postmenopausal woman is to go forth and reseed the
> community with her concentrated kernel of truth and wisdom. In
> some native cultures, menopausal women were felt to retain their "wise
> blood," rather than shed it cyclically, and were therefore considered
> more powerful than menstruating women. A woman could not be a
> shaman until she was past menopause in these cultures.
>
> —Christiane Northrup, M.D.

Menopause is a natural process comprised of three stages. Around the age of
forty, the amount of estrogen produced by the ovaries begins to decline. By
the age of forty-seven or so, a woman enters perimenopause, where periods
become less consistent. Menopause, from the Greek *month* and *pause*, occurs
when monthly bleeding stops altogether. The third stage, postmenopause, occurs after a year with no menstrual bleeding.

A woman's experience of the change of life is as individual as she is. Factors
such as expectation, diet, stress, emotional support, self-esteem, and heredity
play important roles. For women who cherish the Seven Treasures and practice Hatha Yoga throughout their lives, the difficulties of menopause are notably
less intense. Still, as the body adjusts to the rapidly changing chemical balance,
some physical discomfort may be experienced, even by active, healthy, positive
women. The symptoms encountered are usually attributed to an imbalance of
vata, or wind, from an Ayurvedic perspective. As we enter our later years, our
bodies have a natural tendency to dry out. Stress, anxiety, and general scurrying
around have a similar effect that meets us head-on through this time of energetic
and hormonal adjustment. This is not a time for guilt trips. It is, however, a time
to check in with your level of vital reserves. If you've been pushing yourself for
years, try to change course before your estrogen levels fall. Give your adrenal
and other glands a chance to recover from their exhausted state. Rejuvenate and
replenish what you can through the Seven Treasures and regular yoga practice.

Yoga *asana* practice has a unique stabilizing effect on hormonal imbalances
in general.

Explore these practices as regular additions to your life as you enter the menopausal years. Modify them accordingly and insert them into a basic practice. Note their effect on your moods and irritability. They will support your nervous and glandular systems.

Practices for Menopause

1. Spread Leg Forward Fold Pose (*Prasarita Padottanasana*)

2. Standing Forward Fold Pose (*Uttanasana*)

3. Downward-Facing Dog Pose (*Adho Mukha Shvanasana*)

4. Head-to-Knee Pose (*Janu Shirshasana*)—Forward

5. Posterior Stretch Pose (*Paschimottanasana*)

6. Inverted Action Pose (*Viparita Karani*) or Shoulder Stand Pose (*Sarvangasana*) or any Supported Inversion Pose

7. Plow Pose (*Halasana*)

8. Half Fish Pose (*Ardha Matsyasana*) or Supported Fish Pose—Make It Easier version

9. Head Stand Pose (*Shirshasana*)

10. Optimal Diaphragmatic Breathing (not pictured; see page 156)

11. *Ujjayi* Breathing (not pictured; see page 159)

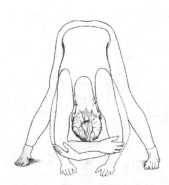

Spread Leg Forward Pose

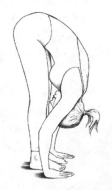

Standing Forward Fold Pose

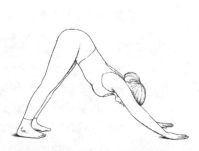

Downward-Facing Dog Pose

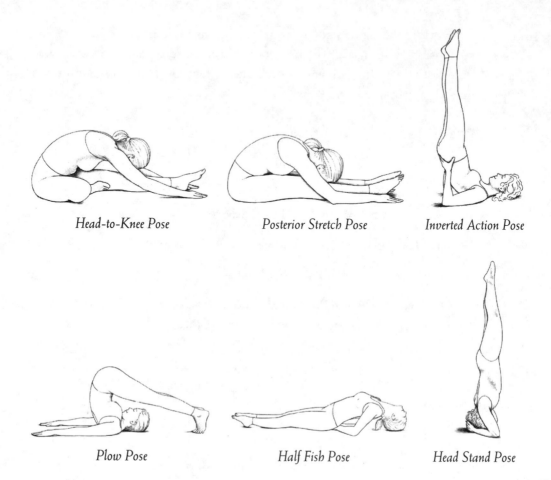

Head-to-Knee Pose   Posterior Stretch Pose   Inverted Action Pose

Plow Pose   Half Fish Pose   Head Stand Pose

12. Alternate Nostril Breathing (*Nadi Shodhanam*) (not pictured; see page 159)

13. For countering hot flashes and night sweats or irritability, use any of the first five poses above and Optimal Diaphragmatic Breathing.

BONE HEALTH AND OSTEOPOROSIS

When we learn to move as infants, the fundamentals we master are pushing, grasping, and pulling actions. This puts us into interaction with gravity and with people and things in our environment. Through movement, we learn to satisfy our curiosity and get our needs met. As we enter our later years, we must not be lured into Western culture's gluttony for luxury. Bone health requires that we continue to physically assert ourselves in our world.

By the age of thirty-five, our bodies reach their peak bone mass, which is when bones are strongest. After this time, bones gradually lose their density until menopause, when the loss accelerates by as much as 3 percent per year. This rapid loss is directly related to the absence of estrogen, which is why osteoporosis affects many more women than men. Healthy bones are acquired through a healthful lifestyle, balanced diet, and exercise when young. Bone loss later in life and after menopause can be slowed down the same way it is built up in youth. A calcium- and vitamin D-rich diet is essential. From age thirty-five on, you should have at least 1,000 milligrams of calcium in your diet daily. Some research recommends as much as 1,500 milligrams of calcium per day from a bio-available source such as calcium citrate or calcium carbonate if you're not taking estrogen. Lowfat dairy foods, leafy greens, nuts, and seeds are good dietary sources of calcium. Reduce your intake of colas, as they contain phosphate, which interferes with calcium absorption; and limit caffeine, as it increases the rate at which you excrete calcium and other minerals in your urine.

A yoga practice that builds strength and improves flexibility, agility, and balance gives you an edge against osteoporosis. When you're strong, flexible, agile, and have good balance, you're less likely to fall and less likely to break something if you do. One study by Miriam Nelson at Tufts University showed that when muscle mass increased through strength training in postmenopausal women, their bone density increased as well. Not only did they not lose bone mass like the control group, these women added it!

To support bone health, put these strengthening practices into your routine, and be sure to interact often with gravity in some aerobic way!

1. Chair Pose (*Utkatasana*)

2. Powerful Pose (*Ugrasana*)

3. Dynamic Warrior Pose 1 or 2 (*Virabhadrasana Vinyasa Krama* 1 or 2)

4. Triangle Pose (*Trikonasana*)

5. King Dancer Pose (*Natarajasana*) or Tree Pose (*Vrikshasana*) or Standing Scale Pose (*Tolasana*)

6. Downward-Facing Dog Pose (*Adho Mukha Shvanasana*)

7. Four-Limb Staff Pose (*Chaturanga Dandasana*)

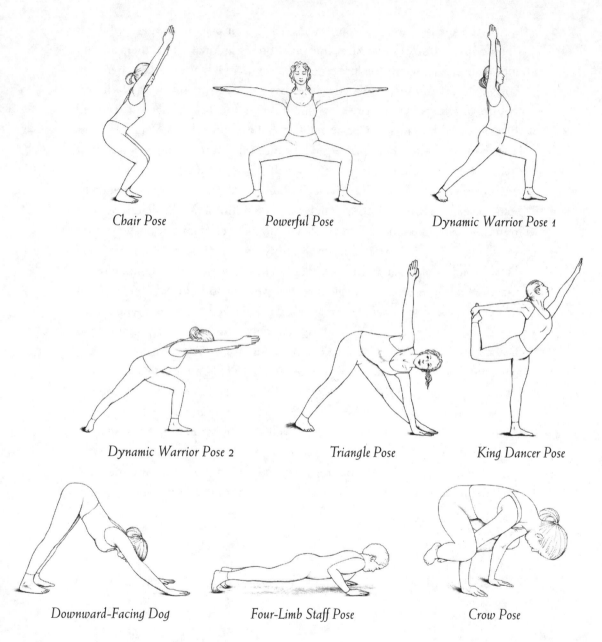

Chair Pose

Powerful Pose

Dynamic Warrior Pose 1

Dynamic Warrior Pose 2

Triangle Pose

King Dancer Pose

Downward-Facing Dog

Four-Limb Staff Pose

Crow Pose

8. Crow Pose (*Bhujapidasana*)

9. Upward-Facing Plank Pose (*Purvottanasana*) (pose not pictured; see page 84)

10. Moving Practice—Concept Exploration (not pictured; see chapter 6)

For Concept Exploration, choose a theme that engages you with gravity or with objects that offer some resistance. Here is one possibility. Think of something you care deeply about that might be threatened. Now connect that feeling to power in your arms and legs. Protect it by pressing the threat away. Move according to your feelings. Use the floor and the wall to press against. Feel a connection throughout your body; feel the support of the bones through your arms and legs. Keep pressing with all your strength. Apply the Root Lock (*Mula Bandha*) and continue. Find your will to live and press with that in mind. Use any image that supports your right to be.

Yet another option that is not as intense, and is quite fun, is to buy a rebounder or mini-trampoline and jump for several minutes each day. This also supports your cellular metabolism. Also useful is walking while moving hand weights in different ways around your body. (I do this early in the morning when very few people in my neighborhood are awake so they won't see me gesticulating with arm weights. I also wear a small weight belt.)

BREAST CARE

The Seven Treasures in chapter 12, combined with regular Hatha Yoga, keep the glandular balance of the breast tissue as harmonious as possible over the child-bearing years. From the point of view of posture practice, keeping the chest muscles strong will support the breasts. If you're looking for this, incorporate the Four-Limb Staff Pose (*Chaturanga Dandasana*) and the Downward-Facing Dog Pose (*Adho Mukha Shvanasana*), both of which can be done in the Sun Salutation. You may also wish to walk with weights or add upper-body weight training to your overall fitness plan. The Fish Pose (*Matsyasana*) offers opening to the chest region and circulation to the mammary glands, which is especially useful during breast-feeding. Hydrating and ensuring regular bowel movements will help keep the lymphatic and glandular tissues in this area flowing.

Because the incidence of breast cancer is currently so high, I am including a brief program for recovery from the tightness and loss of range of motion that follows a mastectomy and radiation therapy. The practice can help reintegrate the use of the affected chest and arm areas.

Practices for Recovery from Treatment of Breast Cancer

1. Desk Pose (*Dvipada Pitham*)

2. Universal Twist Pose (*Shava Udarakarshanasana*)

3. Twist to Flapping Fish Posture Loop (*Shava Udarakarshanasana* to *Matsya Kridasana Vinyasa Krama*)

4. Abdominal Stretch Pose (*Jathara Parivritta*) (pose not pictured; see page 74)

5. Cobra Pose (*Bhujangasana*), Versions 1 and 2

6. Sitting Side Bend Pose (*Parshvottanasana*), and with arm wrapped behind

7. Upward-Facing Plank Pose (*Purvottanasana*)

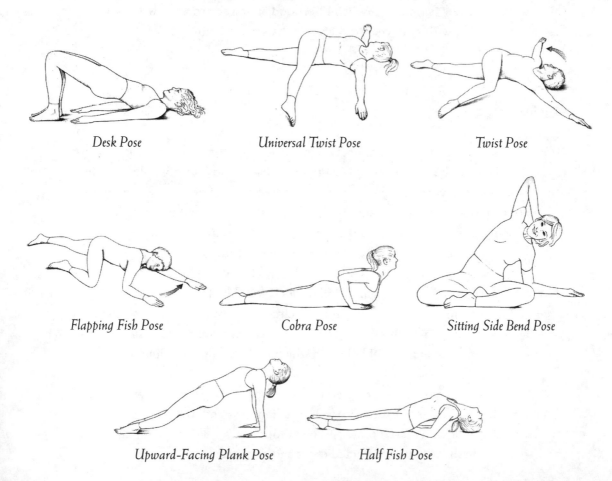

Desk Pose   *Universal Twist Pose*   *Twist Pose*

Flapping Fish Pose   *Cobra Pose*   *Sitting Side Bend Pose*

Upward-Facing Plank Pose   *Half Fish Pose*

8. Half Fish Pose (*Ardha Matsyasana*)—Make It Easier variation

9. Healing *Pranayama* (not pictured; see page 157)

10. Vocalization (not pictured; see page 162)

11. Moving Practice—Remedial Movement (not pictured; see page 146)

For Remedial Movement, mobility and strength are integrated as you move objects in all dimensions around your torso. Make up a dynamic practice by using your arms to move dowels, a broom, soup cans, or ten-ounce water bottles. Don't just move them up and down or in and out. Make big curlicues, figure eights, zigzags near and far. Make intricate spatial forms so you can recover the use of every possible cell to full functioning and get *prana* coursing through the affected tissues.

If you're undergoing treatment for breast cancer, Optimal Diaphragmatic Breathing is of help. Healing *pranayama* helps restore and distribute your vitality, and it doesn't take much effort—just breathing and thinking, and you're doing that anyway! My yoga students and associates who have been through treatment confirm that the following *pranayama* practices are valuable in coping with fear and anxiety:

❋ 2-to-1 Ratioed Breathing

❋ *Ujjayi* Breathing

❋ Alternate Nostril Breathing (*Nadi Shodhanam*)

❋ Vocalization

INCONTINENCE

Incontinence can occur at any time, but happens to many women after childbirth, after prolonged illness, or as we become more sedentary. To prevent and possibly rectify incontinence and pelvic organ prolapse, add these practices on a regular basis.

Caution: Avoid all practices that apply strong downward pressure.

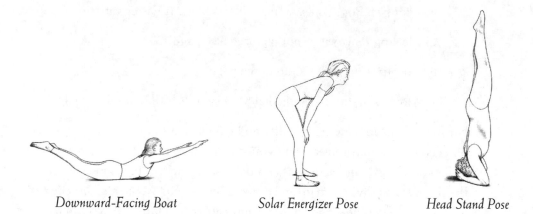

Downward-Facing Boat   *Solar Energizer Pose*   *Head Stand Pose*

1. Downward-Facing Boat Pose (*Adho Mukha Navasana*)

2. Solar Energizer with emphasis on Root Lock (*Agni Sara* with *Mula Bandha*). You may do this practice lying on your back.

3. Choose any of these inverted poses: Head Stand Pose (*Shirshasana*), Inverted Action Pose (*Viparita Karani*), Shoulder Stand Pose (*Sarvangasana*), Supported Inversion Poses (Versions 1, 2, or 3)

fire, flow, and a healthy glow: energy issues

Yoga is a very practical system based on fundamental natural laws. A simple engine requires a regulated flow of fuel and ignition to produce heat and work. Our bodies are sustained energetically in a similar way. Ancient texts describe three vital essences as the components of our life engine. They are *prana*, *tejas*, and *ojas* (see the table on the following page).

Prana, the life force, possesses the characteristic of flow. Yoga practices pump *prana* in specific ways throughout the body through subtle channels called *nadis*. The flow of *prana* can be aggravated or diminished overall or in different areas. This is an important feature in energy maintenance. With anything that flows, the question becomes one of regulating the amount. *Pranic* force can surge and pool or become blocked and reduced to a trickle, creating problems in either case. Of Ayurveda's three humors (*doshas*), *prana* corresponds to *vata*, the combination of ether and air elements.

Table 8.1 The three vital essences

Vital Essence	Relates to	Dosha	Function	Associated with
Prana		Vata	flow	vital force, breath, *chi*, spirit
Tejas		Pitta	fire	metabolic fire, *agni*, transformation
Ojas		Kapha	fuel	vigor, *jing*, life sap, cohesion

Pranic flow stokes the central bodily fire (*agni*) at the solar plexus, which ignites the furnace of digestion and assimilation of nutrients. With a strong digestive fire, our engine runs clean, transforming fuel into energy and heat. When *agni* is weak, food components are no longer adequately digested and cannot be absorbed. We lose power and accumulate waste. Foods that are fresh and close to their natural state burn cleaner than highly processed or preserved foods because they are filled with *prana* and leave little residue (*ama*).

Spread throughout the body, the second essence, *tejas*, is the more subtle level of *agni*, further transforming nourishment into power and light. Ayurvedic physician Vasant Lad writes that *tejas* governs metabolism through the enzyme system. (Enzymes are catalysts to chemical changes in the body.) I experience *tejas* as heat and light emanating from the mitochondria, which are the cellular powerhouses. This concurs with its definition as the glow of healthy cellular metabolism. *Tejas* walks the line between physical substance and subtle force, inciting transformation at every level of our being. Of Ayurveda's three humors, *tejas* corresponds to *pitta*, the fire element.

The third subtle essence, *ojas*, is the refined yield of all the body tissues (the seven *dhatus*). It is distilled at each hierarchical level of tissue formation, resulting in a potent life sap that functions as the foundation of our immunity. Of Ayurveda's three humors, *ojas* corresponds to *kapha*, the substantial combination of water and earth elements. The abundance of *ojas* depends on the equipoise between *prana* and *tejas*. Vibrant health and radiant beauty are outward signs that the three subtle essences are balanced, abundant, and flowing.

At the most fundamental level, health issues concerning energy revolve around these three essences. For thousands of years before the invention of Prozac, people were using yogic and Ayurvedic methods to cleanse and nourish the body and to restore the balance of these essential elements of life.

VITALITY AND LONGEVITY

The signs of our lifestyle choices stand out in our health as we get older. I'm sure you've seen people who look ten or twenty years older than their age, and also the fortunate ones who look much younger. Each person acquires an amount of *ojas* (life sap) at birth. We retain this basic vitality and invest in longevity by living a balanced, wholesome life. If we squander our vital essence through depleting activities, it's like punching holes in a paper cup filled with water—our life juice drains out. Then when faced with an emergency or disease, our resistance is compromised.

Factors that disrupt our three vital essences (*prana, tejas,* and *ojas*) are poor diet, smoking, alcohol and drug use, poor digestion and elimination, irregular routine, lack of sleep, overwork, lack of or too much exercise, mental anguish, worry and anxiety, and emotional imbalance of any sort. Welcome to modern living! Of course, factors beyond our control, such as viruses, trauma, and injury, take their toll as well. We can do our best to retain and restore vigor through yogic methods that shore up our ability to withstand and counter the effects of harmful factors.

live "juicy" with these daily rejuvenators

- Natural oil massage and sufficient oil in your diet protects you from dryness (withering).
- Juicy food (such as soups), juicy fruits (such as melons, grapes, and berries), and vegetables keep your tissues moist. Eat life to retain and restore life.
- Water, herbal tea, fresh vegetable juice, and fruit juice are good drink choices. (Water the juice down, half water/half juice, for fewer calories.) Coffee is drying, so if you drink it, drink water, too (and take a calcium supplement).
- Include aerobic movement, preferably outdoors in sunlight, for *pranic* recharge, cleansing, and flow.
- Take 5—Just rest for a few moments, focus on the breath, and let go of your concerns. Relaxation and meditation cleanse the mind and nourish the soul.

These practices are not a quick fix. Depending on what your lifestyle is, it may take weeks or months for you to notice consistent results. When you do, you'll find that they are quite remarkable and will spur you on. Keeping yoga practice going in your life requires commitment and awareness as you refine your ability to self-regulate. The resulting vitality, stamina, beauty, self-control, and confidence are well worth the effort. Pay attention to cleansing and dietary awareness, as they are essential.

What we're after here is a posture practice that engages your mind and will with an appropriate challenge, gives you a light cleansing sweat, stokes *agni*, moves *prana* through every part of your body, and massages the internal organs. Here is one such routine. Be sure to choose the versions of the recommended poses that suit your needs right now. Once you understand in your body the effects of these postures in relation to the goal of the practice, alter your program with additional postures.

Two practice routines are suggested. The first one is for restoration. If you're presently in a debilitated state, follow this one until you've recovered more energy. Take time for inner exploration. Get help with habit patterns as needed. There are wonderful retreat programs around the world that can help you get a leg up on making initial changes in your health habits.

The second practice is vigorous. It gives you the most bang for your buck. Use it to carefully power up your reserves. But beware. I've seen advanced practitioners literally burn out through practice by overkindling their fire and burning up *ojas*. Be consistent in your practice, but don't overtrain. Take time off or vary your routine with an occasional restorative practice. You'll come back stronger!

If you're suffering from low energy, look to your diet and seek guidance for more focused tissue cleansing.

Restorative Practice

1. Solar Energizer (*Agni Sara*)

2. Abdominal Stretch Pose (*Jathara Parivritta*) or Half Moon Pose (*Ardha Chandrasana*)

3. Cobra Pose (*Bhujangasana*)

4. Universal Twist Pose (*Shava Udarakarshanasana*)

5. Posterior Stretch Pose (*Paschimottanasana*) or Make It Easier with Support

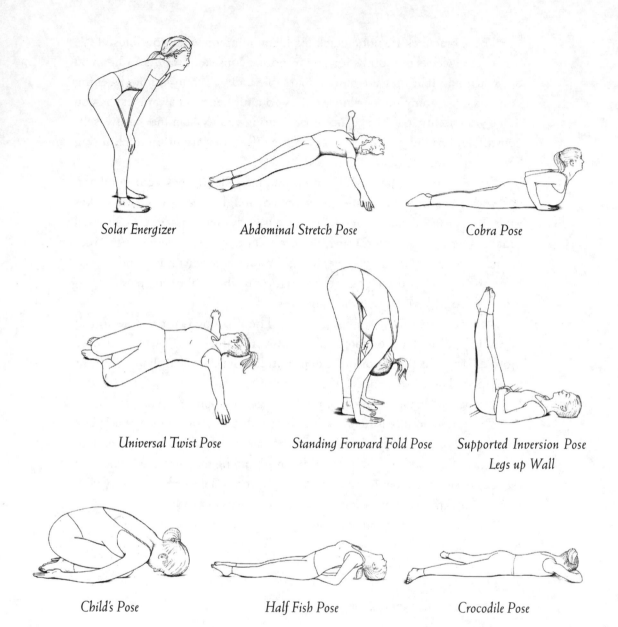

Solar Energizer

Abdominal Stretch Pose

Cobra Pose

Universal Twist Pose

Standing Forward Fold Pose

Supported Inversion Pose
Legs up Wall

Child's Pose

Half Fish Pose

Crocodile Pose

6. Standing Forward Fold Pose (*Uttanasana*) or Spread Leg Forward Fold Pose (*Prasarita Padottanasana*)

7. Wind-Eliminating Pose (*Supta Pavanamuktasana*) (pose not pictured, see page 115)

8. Supported Inversion Poses: Feet on Chair, Legs up Wall, or the Perfect Wedge

9. Child's Pose (*Balasana*)

10. Supported Half Fish Pose (*Matsyasana*)

11. Crocodile Pose (*Makarasana*) and/or Flapping Fish Pose (*Matsya Kridasana*) for deep relaxation and breath awareness

Power-Up Practice

1. Solar Energizer (*Agni Sara*)

2. Upward-Facing Boat Pose Series (*Navasana*): Choose any (poses not pictured; see page 45)

3. Locust Pose (*Shalabhasana*) or Half Locust Pose (*Ardha Shalabhasana*)

4. Choose from Warrior Pose (*Virabhadrasana*), Chair Pose (*Utkatasana*), Powerful Pose (*Ugrasana*), or do them all!

5. Abdominal Twist Pose (*Jathara Parivartanasana*) or Double Leg Lift with Solar Energizer (*Utthita Dvipadasana* with *Agni Sara*)

6. Downward-Facing Dog Pose (*Adho Mukha Shvanasana*)

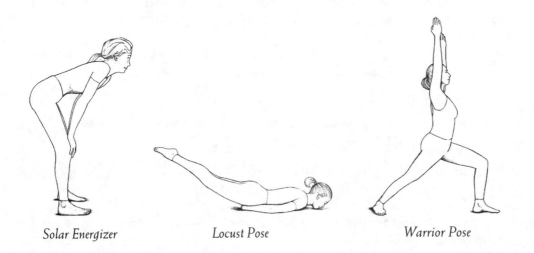

Solar Energizer   *Locust Pose*   *Warrior Pose*

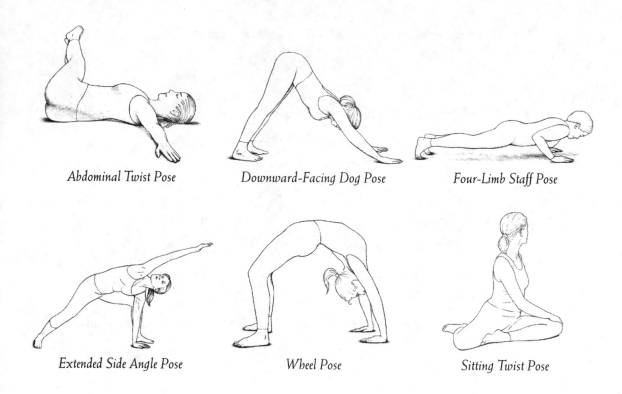

Abdominal Twist Pose   Downward-Facing Dog Pose   Four-Limb Staff Pose

Extended Side Angle Pose   Wheel Pose   Sitting Twist Pose

7. Four-Limb Staff Pose (*Chaturanga Dandasana*)

8. Choose from Head-to-Knee Pose (*Janu Shirshasana*)—Side, or Extended Side Angle Pose (*Utthita Parsvakonasana*).

9. Cobra Pose (*Bhujangasana*) as preparation for Bow Pose (*Dhanurasana*), Half Bow Pose (*Ardha Dhanurasana*), or Wheel Pose (*Chakrasana*)

10. Choose from Sitting Twist Pose (*Bharadvajasana*), Spinal Twist Pose (*Matsyendrasana*), Half Spinal Twist Pose (*Ardha Matsyendrasana*), or Side Angle Twist Pose (*Parivritta Parshvakonasana*)

11. Wind-Eliminating Pose (*Supta Pavanamuktasana*) (pose not pictured; see page 115)

12. Head-to-Knee Pose (*Janu Shirshasana*)—Forward, or Posterior Stretch Pose (*Paschimottanasana*)

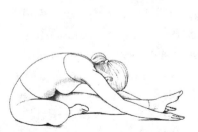

Head-to-Knee Pose—Forward

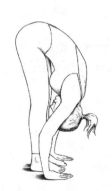

Standing Forward Fold Pose

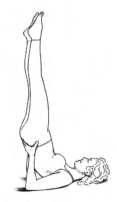

Inverted ActionPose

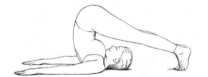

Plow Pose

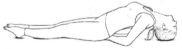

Half Fish Pose

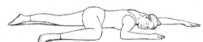

Flapping Fish Pose

13. Standing Forward Fold Pose (*Uttanasana*) or Spread Leg Forward Fold Pose (*Prasarita Padottanasana*)

14. Inverted Action Pose (*Viparita Karani*), Shoulder Stand Pose (*Sarvangasana*), or Supported Inversion Poses: Legs on Chair, Feet up Wall, or The Perfect Wedge

15. Plow Pose (*Halasana*)

16. Half Fish Pose (*Ardha Matsyasana*)

17. Flapping Fish Pose (*Matsya Kridasana*) and/or Crocodile Pose (*Makarasana*) for deep relaxation and breath awareness

SEXUAL DESIRE AND EXPRESSION

Our fast-paced, hard-driving culture shows up in the bedroom. We manipulate our nervous system with caffeine and other stimulants, and use alcohol and other depressants to come off the caffeine, destroying our natural rhythm for exertion and recuperation. A psychophysical state of stress is not only depleting, but it is a far cry from the open responsiveness conducive to a satisfying sensual relationship. The same culture that created this off-kilter lifestyle offers drugs as a remedy that, in fact, carry us further from our own truth. For many women, childbirth and the responsibility, level of commitment, time, and energy involved in caring for a family are at times overwhelming and draining—even under the best of circumstances. After all the needs have been met, we may have nothing left at the end of the day.

As I discussed earlier, our body naturally dries up and we become less juicy as we age. The seven tissues of the body (*dhatus*) develop in sequence, each formed from the preceding tissue. The first tissue, plasma (*rasa*) is the nutrient-rich base of our blood. *Rasa* means juice. We need to have plentiful, pure, well-nourished juice in order to nourish the final tissue, which is the reproductive tissue (*shukra*). Aphrodisiacs were not always concerned with excitation but rather with easily assimilated *nutrition* to produce high-octane juice! (Such an aphrodisiac could be made of milk, clarified butter, honey, and almonds.) Yet so many women shun nourishment for the sake of fitting into the current cultural mandate of thinness.

Along with a stereotypic image of what makes a woman sexy, our culture also promotes a norm for sexual behavior. We are individuals and our sexuality is very much a part of our personal expression in the world. I think it's tragic when women's magazines and TV shows offering help to women presume that all women want the same level of frequency, intensity, or kind of sexual relations. Your yoga practice will support you in being exactly who you are.

If you're currently in a depleted state, use the restorative practice above until your energy returns. If you're preparing for pregnancy, see that section. Here is another option designed for opening to balanced sexual expression.

A Practice for Balanced Sexual Expression

1. Sun Salutation (*Surya Namaskara*) (pose not pictured; see appendix E)

2. Root Lock (*Mula Bandha*) and Solar Energizer (*Agni Sara*)

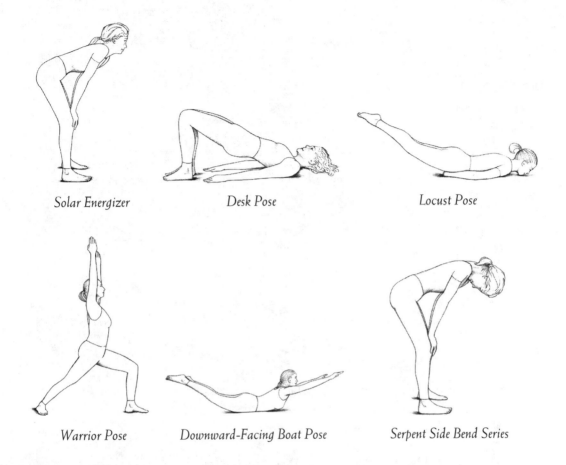

Solar Energizer   Desk Pose   Locust Pose

Warrior Pose   Downward-Facing Boat Pose   Serpent Side Bend Series

3. Desk Pose (*Dvipada Pitham*) or Bridge Pose (*Setu Bandhasana*)

4. Upward-Facing Boat Pose (*Navasana*), any version (pose not pictured; see page 45)

5. Locust Pose (*Shalabhasana*)

6. Warrior Pose (*Virabhadrasana*)

7. Downward-Facing Boat Pose (*Adho Mukha Navasana*)

8. Serpent Side Bend Series (*Anantasana*)

9. Twist to Flapping Fish Posture Loop (*Shava Udarakarshanasana* to *Matsya Kridasana Vinyasa Krama*) (pose not pictured; see page 81)

10. Bow Pose (*Dhanurasana*)

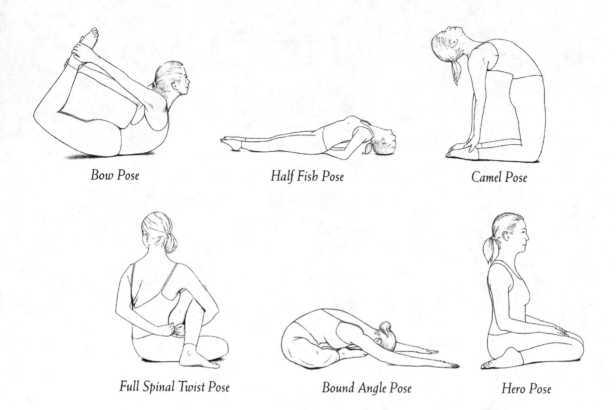

Bow Pose   Half Fish Pose   Camel Pose

Full Spinal Twist Pose   Bound Angle Pose   Hero Pose

11. Half Moon Pose (*Ardha Chandrasana*) (pose not pictured; see page 80)

12. Half Fish Pose (*Ardha Matsyasana*)

13. Camel Pose (*Ushtrasana*) or Wheel Pose (*Chakrasana*)

14. Full Spinal Twist Pose (*Matsyendrasana*)

15. Bound Angle Pose (*Baddha Konasana*) or Reclined Bound Angle Pose (*Supta Baddha Konasana*)

16. Hero Pose (*Virasana*)

17. Spread Leg Forward Fold Pose (*Prasarita Padottanasana*) or Spread Leg Pose (*Upavishtha Konasana*)

18. Child's Pose (*Balasana*)

19. Shoulder Stand Pose (*Sarvangasana*) or Inverted Action Pose (*Vipasta Karani*) (pose not pictured; see page 122)

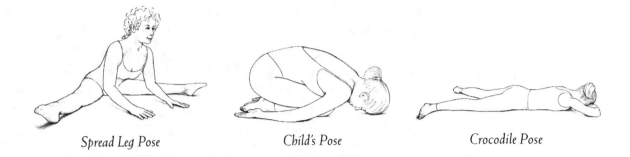

Spread Leg Pose   *Child's Pose*   *Crocodile Pose*

20. Crocodile Pose (*Makarasana*) for deep relaxation

21. Sitting Meditation

22. 2-to-1 Ratioed Breathing (not pictured; see page 157)

23. *Kapalabhati Pranayama* (not pictured; see page 161)

DIGESTION AND ELIMINATION

Roberta, a woman of great stature matched by a boisterous sense of humor, came to me for help with constipation and digestion at the advice of her sister, Renee (who has been in my class for years). Roberta looked matter of fact as we worked our way through the in-take questionnaire, but could no longer contain her sense of disbelief when I demonstrated the yoga postures I was giving her to practice. "Are you nuts?" she blurted out, smiling. "I take antacid and eat so much Ex-Lax my kids think it's candy. You think this is going to do any good?"

Renee said flatly, "It will if you *do it.*"

With an additional promise to drink more water, Roberta left. A few months later, she appeared in my beginning class. Looking great and not as puffy around the eyes, she joked noisily in the back with another student. When we got to the practice of Agni Sara, which I introduce as the most important practice for the digestive system, she blasted from her new yoga mat, "I'll drink to that! I'll drink water any way!" I asked her how that was going, and like the perfect TV commercial testimonial, she told the class, "I didn't believe it either, but since I started this, I don't use laxatives any more, I eat what I want, and I'm still moved every day!"

Proper digestion and elimination are the bedrock of health. Whether or not we are nourished by what we take in depends on our ability to differentiate and assimilate. This is true physically, as well as mentally and emotionally. Time is necessary for complete processing of experiences and events. But we also need an agent of transformation, fire, so that we can assimilate what we've consumed. In addition, we need to be able to release ourselves from things we no longer need through *apana prana*, the downward-flowing force of the body's expulsion. The practices given here are to build *agni*, the fire of transformation, and support *apana prana*. You may need time to withdraw with little stimulation to permit mental and emotional digestion. Take a brisk walk outdoors in clean air. Go alone and allow your mind to clear. Regular meditation practice also gives you a daily retreat into your Self.

Fire-Building *Apana*-Supporting Practice

1. Solar Energizer (*Agni Sara*)

2. Upward-Facing Boat Pose (*Navasana*) (pose not pictured; see page 45)

3. Chair Pose (*Utkatasana*)

4. Powerful Pose (*Ugrasana*)

5. Locust Pose (*Shalabhasana*)

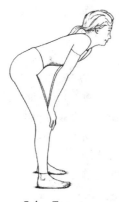

Solar Energizer

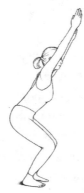

Chair Pose

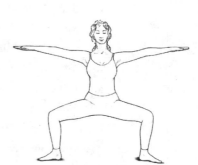

Powerful Pose

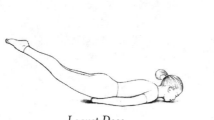

Locust Pose

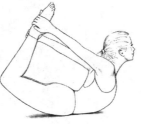

Bow Pose

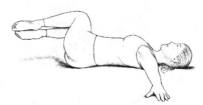

Abdominal Twist Pose, Knees Bent

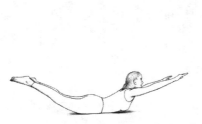

Downward-Facing Boat Pose

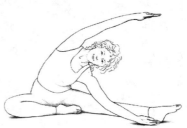

Head-to-Knee Pose

6. Bow Pose (*Dhanurasana*)

7. Double Leg Lift with Solar Energizer (*Utthita Dvipadasana* with *Agni Sara*) (pose not pictured; see page 56)

8. Abdominal Twist Pose (*Jathara Parivartanasana*)

9. Downward-Facing Boat Pose (*Adho Mukha Navasana*)

10. Head-to-Knee Pose (*Janu Shirshasana*)—Side

11. Monkey Pose (*Banarasana*)

12. Abdominal Stretch Pose (*Jathara Parivritta*) (pose not pictured; see page 74)

13. Hero Pose (*Virasana*)

14. Sitting Twist Pose (*Bharadvajasana*)

15. Revolved Triangle Pose (*Parivritta Trikonasana*)

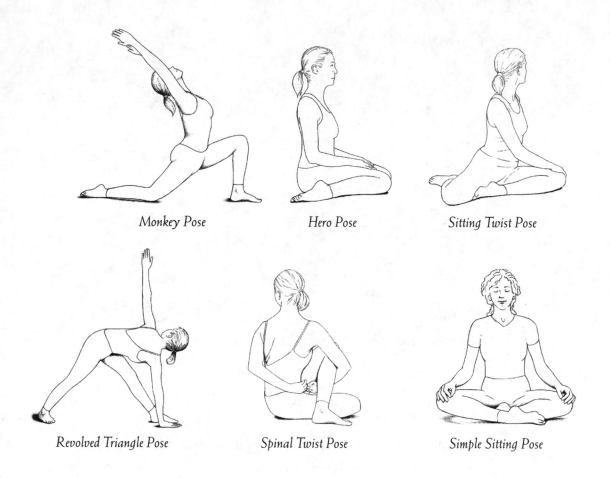

Monkey Pose   Hero Pose   Sitting Twist Pose

Revolved Triangle Pose   Spinal Twist Pose   Simple Sitting Pose

16. Spinal Twist Pose (*Matsyendrasana*)

17. Symbol of Yoga (*Yoga Mudrasana*) (pose not pictured; see page 106)

18. Simple Sitting Pose (*Sukhasana*) for relaxation practice

FATIGUE

When you're fatigued, it probably seems obvious that you need rest. The so-lution could certainly be this easy. May I suggest a natural retreat setting for R&R rather than a stressful vacation scene with unhealthy food and question-able recuperative value? (See appendix C for suggestions on where to go.) However, sometimes rest alone doesn't do the trick. We may be fatigued because we don't receive enough nourishment or we may not be able to use what we're taking in because something is awry in our ability to process. Or we may be blocked somewhere down the line, with things backing up. We have to address fatigue individually and discern which attributes of our energy use are not functioning well. We can begin with an analysis of some important aspects of health.

Nourishment. Look to your diet. Are you living on Diet Pepsi and no-fat pretzels? Or nutritionally empty donuts and coffee? And how do you eat—standing over the kitchen counter while you're cooking for everyone else? What about your relationships? Are you a giver and not a receiver? Do you take time for yourself? Have you had a relaxing bath lately, been for a walk in the park, seen the sun set? Deeply satisfying experiences are nourishing as well.

Processing. Take a solitary walk in sunlight to stimulate your physical and mental digestion. Take someone along only if they're willing to process with you. You don't want more information or disturbing input. *Agni Sara* and the practices I've given for digestion and elimination will help on the physical level. Try Concept Exploration from chapter 6, "The Essential Moving Practices for Women," with the theme of taking in and letting go. How do you respond to this theme? How does it feel in your body? What movements happen and what are the feelings that go with them?

Unblocking. Whether the place where you're stuck is physical, emotional, or mental, moving your *prana* is the way to get unstuck. Experiment with these practical suggestions. Try the Restorative Practice under the Vitality and Longevity section early in this chapter and see whether you feel more energized or more lethargic afterward. If you feel worse after it, then try this gently stimulating option: Track your experience and watch how you feel after

ginger improves the power of your digestion

Ginger root is an excellent natural aid to digestion because it improves appetite, stimulates *agni* (digestive fire), and reduces *ama* (waste). Add it to your cooking in fresh or powdered form or make ginger tea. It's simple. Just boil water, pour into your cup, and add a thin slice or two of fresh ginger. Let it steep for three to five minutes, remove ginger slice, and drink.

each pose. Or dance to music you can relate to, no matter how out of vogue it may be. You've done this, right? Shut the door, turn it up, dance, sing, and let the spirit move you. Yoga meets you at every level of your self, so even though these recommendations are physical things to do, use them as metaphors, meaning-filled poetic ventures that give you information about your life.

Gentle Stimulating Practice

1. Sun Salutation (*Surya Namaskara*) (pose not pictured; see appendix E)

2. Extended Triangle Pose (*Utthita Trikonasana*)

3. Tree Pose (*Vrikshasana*)

4. Standing Forward Fold Pose (*Uttanasana*)

5. Crocodile Pose (*Makarasana*)

6. Cobra Pose (*Bhujangasana*)

7. Child's Pose (*Balasana*)

8. Sitting Twist Pose (*Bharadvajasana*)

9. Bound Angle Pose (*Baddha Konasana*)

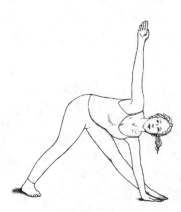

Extended Triangle Pose

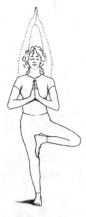

Tree Pose

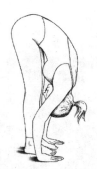

Standing Forward Fold

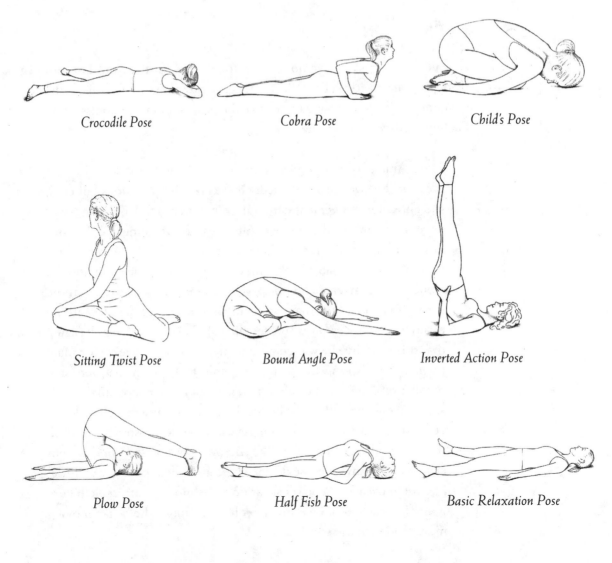

Crocodile Pose

Cobra Pose

Child's Pose

Sitting Twist Pose

Bound Angle Pose

Inverted Action Pose

Plow Pose

Half Fish Pose

Basic Relaxation Pose

10. Inverted Action Pose (*Viparita Karani*) or Shoulder Stand (*Sarvangasana*)

11. Plow Pose (*Halasana*)

12. Half Fish Pose (*Ardha Matsyasana*)

13. Basic Relaxation Pose (*Shavasana*)

14. Healing *Pranayama* in Basic Relaxation Pose (pose not pictured; see page 129)

DEPRESSION

As a yoga therapist, I have no rote protocol, save for the truth I experience through yoga practice. This allows me to be present in interaction with each client during our session and to observe the process of interaction as it unfolds. Each person's work is unique.

> Mary Ann, a former yoga student, came to me to work on her depression. She was also under a doctor's care. Of the options I offered, she chose free movement exploration practice. The only thing was, once we began, she didn't move. After years of watching people move in structured, semi-structured and fully open ways, I had never witnessed someone in absolute stillness for more than a few minutes, let alone three-quarters of an hour! My own insecurity insisted that she try a different tack, perhaps some invigorating *pranayama* (breathing practices) or *vinyasa krama* (posture flows). She declined, emphasizing that this was why she was coming to me. So we met weekly for a fall, a winter, and a spring. She would lie comfortably on my mat, very still, hardly breathing, and I would watch her. But I would more than watch her—I would be with her fully for that hour, as present as I could be, yet human and distracted as I am. As winter turned to spring, I noticed that her body seemed fuller, like she was more puffed up, more energized somehow. The next time she came, she moved, just a little, like the movements you see a cat do to be more comfortable before going back to sleep. Over the next few meetings, she began moving more, and then the words came.

The word *yoga* means union, and it refers fundamentally to the union of the individual drop of a soul with the vast ocean of Supreme Consciousness. Every soul's journey is unique, but each has the same ultimate goal: the recollection of belonging. Yoga practices support this subtle shift from identification with the drop-like ego to identification with the Divine on every level of our being. As drops, we already belong in the ocean; our path is to realize this.

Yoga teaches that we become depressed because we're disconnected from our mission of union. We have disconnected at the beginning and at the end. We have unplugged from the yearning, the spark of creativity that drives us through life against daunting odds (the push). And we have withdrawn hope (the reach), the blind optimism that we indeed do belong. The life force, however, thrusts us forward. When we remain connected to our soul's expression in life (*spanda*), no matter how far off the beaten path it takes us, life flows through us. But many times we opt not to ride this sometimes overwhelming and tumultuous current. We solidify around a role or an event in the drama and hold up against the current of life.

On the path of yoga, one learns to view the personality as a collection of mental and emotional habits and usually unconscious behavioral loops. Yoga gives us the option of a higher vantage point. Many approaches aimed at relieving depression try to nudge us out of the groove of mental dullness (*tamas*). Exercise, nature, light, drugs, and visiting people and places from happier days are all attempts to skip the record needle over to a more upbeat song. The double edge of depression is that the song presently playing is the one we need to complete our soul's journey to wholeness. Many conventional Western professionals recommend a multi-angled approach that considers safety, on the one hand, and careful processing, on the other. If you suspect you're depressed, get help from your doctor, counselor, or clergyperson. I offer as an example the program Mary Ann followed.

Mary Ann was under the care of a psychiatrist who agreed that exercise, including yoga, would be good for her. She was taking Prozac and meeting with a counselor weekly. Our work was twofold. She engaged in a moving practice in my presence as described above, which later included verbal dialogue. She also did these practices to support her body during this time of withdrawal.

Mary Ann's Supportive Practice for Time of Withdrawal

1. Sun Salutation (*Surya Namaskara*) (pose not pictured; see appendix E)

2. Warrior Dynamic Pose 1 (*Virabhadrasana Vinyasa Krama 1*) (pose not pictured, see page 54)

3. Standing Forward Fold Pose (*Uttanasana*)

4. Extended Triangle Pose (*Utthita Trikonasana*), Angle Pose (*Konasana*), Revolved Triangle Pose (*Parivritta Trikonasana*) in sequence

5. Downward-Facing Boat Pose (*Adho Mukha Navasana*)

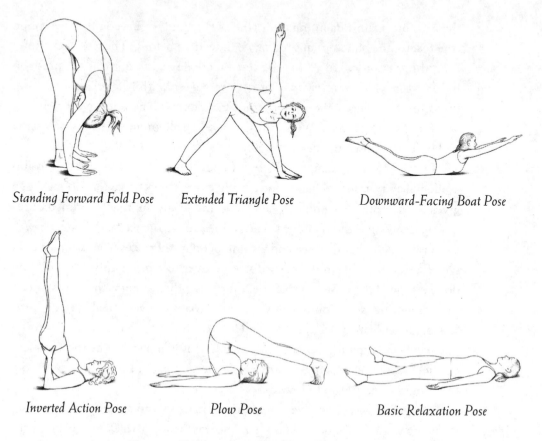

Standing Forward Fold Pose   Extended Triangle Pose   Downward-Facing Boat Pose

Inverted Action Pose   Plow Pose   Basic Relaxation Pose

6. Twist to Flapping Fish Posture Loop (*Shava Udarakarshanasana to Matsya Kridasana Vinyasa Krama*) (pose not pictured; see page 81)

7. Inverted Action Pose (*Viparita Karani*), Plow Pose (*Halasana*), Fish Pose (*Matsyasana*) in sequence

8. Crocodile Pose (*Makarasana*) or Basic Relaxation Pose (*Shavasana*)

beauty

Supermodels and celebrities tout yoga as an essential for a svelte and sexy body. From Madonna's exclusive yoga lessons to sightings of Sara Jessica Parker at Jivamukti to Christy Turlington's famed "yoga butt" (her words, not mine), we deduce that yoga works in the beauty department. But is beauty only the possession of the anatomically blessed? What about the older woman with the confident laugh and irresistible glow? Or the working single mother who seems inexhaustibly perky? Or the medical student who, resistant to her brutal schedule, shows no signs of distress? Yoga develops inner balance, which leads to vibrant health, a by-product of which is physical beauty. The bottom line is, if you practice yoga and hold the Seven Treasures dear, you'll look your personal best!

All you need to boost your radiance quotient is regular basic practice of the following:

❋ Postures (*asanas*)

❋ *Pranayama*, or dynamic practice (*vinyasa karma*) in which *pranayama* is integrated into posture practice

❋ Meditation and/or movement processing

❋ The Seven Treasures of Balanced Health (see chapter 12)

BODY BEAUTIFUL YOGA

To go body beautiful with yoga, you'll need to work gradually into a strengthening, body-shaping practice. But note! The practice your best friend does may not be enough for you or it may exhaust you. You're not stronger or weaker; you're simply different. It's important to remain aware of your own body's needs and to experiment to learn what works for you. Be sure to include the counterposes to balance the work you did in the body-shaping practices. Supplement with some type of aerobic exercise, such as brisk walking. Some advanced yoga practitioners can perform demanding dynamic posture sequences because they train aerobically through yoga practice alone. Applying specific breathing practices and energy recyclers (*bandhas*) would easily thrust these practice sequences into that category. However, because such advanced techniques are not safe for everyone, it would be irresponsible for me to describe them here. Fortunately, finding experienced teachers is much easier these days than ever before. Up until this level, add thirty to forty-five minutes of aerobics to these two practice sequences four or more times a week. You can alternate them for variety, or begin with the first sequence and feed the alternate practices (designated by *) from the second sequence into it until you have a "double" practice. Hold each pose for three breaths in the beginning (adjust according to your need!). See if you would like to work up to a minimum of six breaths in each pose.

If you also lift weights or engage in other sports or physical training, you may need to modify this practice so as not to over-train some area of your body. For example, when I train for the AIDS Ride, a long cycling event, my legs get the workout, so I cut back on standing poses that require the knees to bend and instead focus on my abdominals and upper body. If I don't (I've made this mistake), I over-train my legs and then they can't perform. I then have to take time off to recover, losing ground.

Mix and match this program with your basic practice or others of interest from this book. When you adjust your yoga practice to meet your lifestyle, you'll see it more as a supportive friend who is there for you, not as another tedious item on a "To Do" list.

Body Beautiful Practice 1

1. Sun Salutation (*Surya Namaskara*) (pose not pictured; see appendix E)

2. Solar Energizer (*Agni Sara*)

3. Warrior Pose (*Virabhadrasana*) and Warrior Dynamic Pose 2 (*Virabhadrasana Vinyasa Krama* 2)

4. Chair Pose (*Utkatasana*)

5. Triangle Pose (*Trikonasana*), Angle Pose (*Konasana*), Revolved Triangle Pose (*Parivritta Trikonasana*) in sequence

6. Standing Scale Pose (*Tolasana*)

7. Extended Hand-to-Big-Toe Pose (*Utthita Hasta Padangusthasana*)—Forward

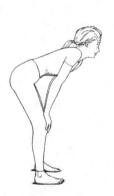

Solar Energizer

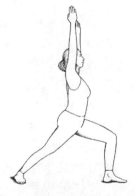

Warrior Pose

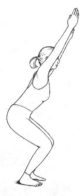

Chair Pose

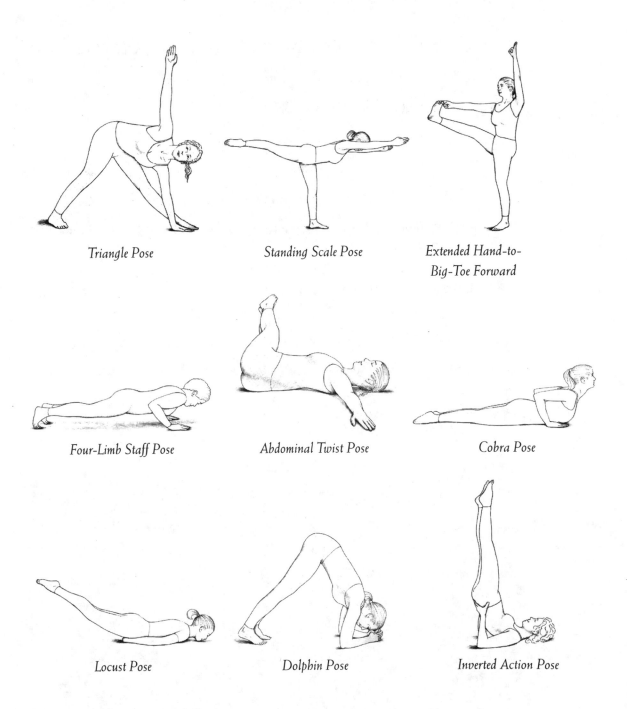

Triangle Pose

Standing Scale Pose

Extended Hand-to-
Big-Toe Forward

Four-Limb Staff Pose

Abdominal Twist Pose

Cobra Pose

Locust Pose

Dolphin Pose

Inverted Action Pose

8. Extended Hand-to-Big-Toe Pose (*Utthita Hasta Padangusthasana*)—Side
(pose not pictured; see page 69)

9. Four-Limb Staff Pose (*Chaturanga Dandasana*)

10. Upward-Facing Boat Pose (*Navasana*) (pose not pictured; see page 45)

11. Abdominal Twist Pose (*Jathara Parivartanasana*)

12. Cobra Pose (*Bhujangasana*)

13. Locust Pose (*Shalabhasana*)

14. Side Plank Pose (*Vasisthasana*) (pose not pictured; see page 63)

15. Dolphin Pose or Scorpion Pose (*Vrishchikasana*)

16. Inverted Action Pose (*Viparita Karani*) or Shoulder Stand Pose (*Sarvangasana*)

Body Beautiful Practice 2

1. Sun Salutation (*Surya Namaskara*) (pose not pictured; see appendix E)

2. Solar Energizer (*Agni Sara*)

3. *Warrior Dynamic Pose 1 and 2 (*Virabhadrasana Vinyasa Krama* 1 and 2)

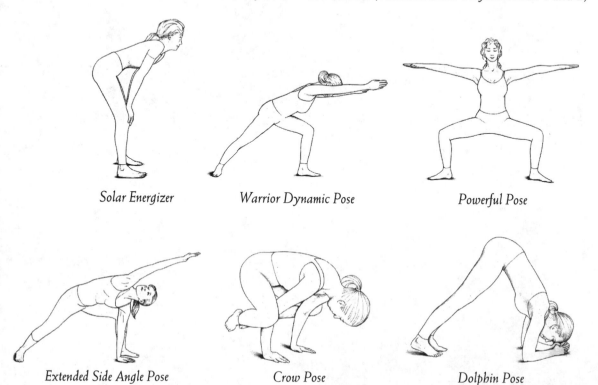

Solar Energizer   Warrior Dynamic Pose   Powerful Pose

Extended Side Angle Pose   Crow Pose   Dolphin Pose

4. *Powerful Pose (*Ugrasana*)

5. *Extended Side Angle Pose (*Utthita Parshvakonasana*)

6. *Side Angle Twist Pose (*Parivritta Parshvakonasana*) (pose not pictured; see page 101)

7. *Crow Pose (*Bhujapidasana*)

8. Four-Limb Staff Pose (*Chaturanga Dandasana*) (pose not pictured; see page 62)

9. Upward-Facing Boat Series (*Navasana*) (pose not pictured; see page 45)

10. *Double Leg Lift with Solar Energizer (*Utthita Dvipadasana* with *Agni Sara*) (pose not pictured; see page 56)

11. *Downward-Facing Boat Pose (*Adho Mukha Navasana*) (pose not pictured; see page 58)

12. Dolphin Pose or Scorpion Pose (*Vrishchikasana*)

13. Shoulder Stand Pose (*Sarvangasana*) or Inverted Action Pose (*Viparita Karani*)

Use as recuperative counter-balancing poses:

1. Sit or stand with elbows crossed in front, clasp one up, one down, clasp behind back

2. Sitting Side Bend (*Parshvottanasana*)

3. Posterior Stretch Pose (*Paschimottanasana*)

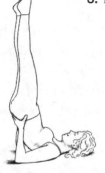
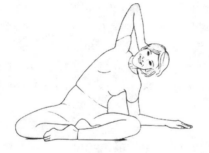
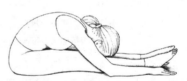

Inverted Action Pose   *Sitting Side Bend*   *Posterior Stretch Pose*

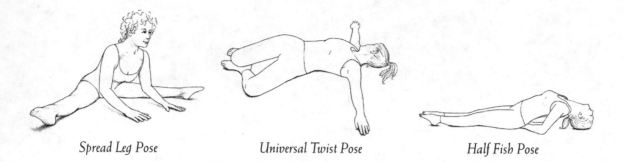

Spread Leg Pose   *Universal Twist Pose*   *Half Fish Pose*

4. Spread Leg Pose (*Upavishtha Konasana*)

5. Universal Twist Pose (*Shava Udarakarshanasana*)

6. Half Fish Pose (*Ardha Matsyasana*)

Feel free to discover other postures to recuperate from the strengthening ones above.

YOGA'S ANTI-AGING ANGLE

If I asked you to visualize an older woman, you would probably describe someone who is withered and wrinkled, hunched over with an uneven gait. As Carrie Demers, M.D., the director of the Center for Health and Healing, writes, "The key to health in general and rejuvenation in particular is an abundant supply of *prana* flowing freely at all levels. And this, in turn, requires that we are cleansed and well-nourished." One of the most important yet neglected things to do to keep *prana* flowing is to move! And one thing that makes it possible for us to continue to move well into our later years is healthy joints. In our visualization, the elderly woman couldn't move easily.

For individuals who exercise, joint injury or disease is commonly what takes them off course. Yoga practice trains you to tune in to finer and finer awareness about what is going on in your body, just like a world-class athlete does. You become able to self-adjust. And you become a more informed fitness consumer. Then you don't treat your own body as if someone else knows it better than you do, as did my client Sara.

Sara is a new client. After raising her family, she decided it was time to take care of herself, so after she waved good-bye to her last college-bound offspring, she signed up for membership at her local gym. She learned how to use the weight machines, rower, and treadmill and was told that the yoga class would be good for her. Sara has quite a powerful dose of determination, so she did everything they told her to do with gusto. She came to me with a pulled hamstring, a shoulder injury, and tightness that she said "wouldn't go away." When I asked her about the yoga, she replied, "I shouldn't have tried it; I wasn't able to do much of it." So we spent the next two sessions undoing what Sara's efforts to get into shape at 50-something did to her. Then together we created a joint-freeing, postural muscle-balancing, whole-body integrative practice that will serve her well in whatever forays she makes back into the world of exercise at her gym. Yes, she's going back. As I mentioned, she was determined.

If you've been sedentary and wish to return to exercise, it's extremely important to condition the connective tissue that holds you together. This tissue runs in, around, across, and through the spaces between your bones (and other places, too). If you're older, it's especially prudent to warm up the connective tissue before attempting more strenuous poses. When focusing on the joints, choose movement (*vinyasa krama*) over a held position for greatest

balancing the joints

Some approaches to joint health strengthen the muscles around a joint, sort of solidifying it. This approach stabilizes the joint but does nothing to create balanced mobility through the joint or the entire body. For example, if your knee was compromised, you'd be asked to strengthen the leg muscles that are attached to it. Joints are often injured through repetitive strain caused by alignment imbalances that result from tension in the body. A more holistic view is to open the places where the body is all stuck together and congested. Through moving posture practice and remedial movement, an individual can re-pattern a more balanced way of using the joint. Then with more functional alignment and awareness in place, strengthening enforces a healthful pattern of use. Through attentive practice, yogis learn to detect such imbalances and prevent or reduce strain. Then when joints move, they do so with little wear and tear. The powerful ingredient is awareness.

benefit. Use the following Gentle Joint Limbering Practice to warm up or use it as your practice in its own right. When my husband travels on business, he uses this practice. It helps him counter the hours of sitting, the stress, and the dietary and time changes without overdoing.

Gentle Joint Limbering Practice

1. Circle your wrists and ankles in both directions.

2. Stretch your arms overhead and lower them three or more times. Try different pathways up and down.

3. Clasp your hands, palms together, overhead and imagine drawing a circle on the ceiling. For more work, make the circle larger and larger. Go both directions three or more times.

4. Swing your arms many times—to your sides across-open, in front up-down, and on diagonals around your body where you please.

5. Circle your arms at the shoulders three or more times, and make figure eights.

6. Roll your shoulders forward and back three or more times, together and alternately.

7. March in place, lifting your knees and arms high. Coordinate these movements with your breath, and lift to different places around your body.

8. Circle your thigh in the hip joint, standing on one leg at a time. Or standing wide, roll your hips in a large, even circle, rolling each way several times.

9. Chop. Clasp the arms overhead, breathe in, and look up. Bend the knees, exhale, and bend forward to chop between the legs. Chop diagonally, ear to outside opposite ankle.

10. Twist to each side. Turn your head, reach your arms around behind you, and allow your trailing heel to come off the floor. Alternate several times.

11. Hang over. Bend your knees. Let the spine fold over from your hips. Let the head and arms dangle. If this is too much stretch, place your

hands or elbows on your knees or thighs. Breathe and relax here. Roll slowly up.

Another step in joint health is basic conditioning, which you can accomplish through a posture practice that matches your ability and is done in a way that doesn't exceed your capacity. However, if you're coming to practice after being sedentary for a long time, include these poses, done *vinyasa krama* style. They will help condition your leg and arm joints. Use the Remedial Movement Practice, part 4: Spinal Focus (from chapter 6), to regain a feeling of the through-line of your entire spine. This will help your alignment in posture practice (and in everything you do!).

Basic Joint Conditioning

1. Dynamic Chair Pose (*Utkatasana Vinyasa Krama*)

2. Powerful Dynamic Pose (*Ugrasana Vinyasa Krama*)

3. Preparation for Crow Pose (*Bhujapidasana*): going into and out of the pose

4. Dolphin Pose—going into and out of the pose

5. Desk Pose (*Dvipada Pitham Vinyasa Krama*)—with attention on rolling up and down through the spine

The corrective practices for individual joints will vary; however, a basic practice including these elements will go a long way. Use Gentle Joint Limbering to warm up.

Antidote for the Hunched Posture of Western Civilization

1. Sun Salutation (*Surya Namaskara*). If you don't want to get to the floor here, just do the arch back, the forward fold with hands on a wall a few feet in front of you (pose not pictured, see appendix E).

2. Monkey Pose (*Banarasana*)

3. Extended Triangle Pose (*Utthita Trikonasana*) (pose not pictured; see page 59)

4. Clasp: One up, one down

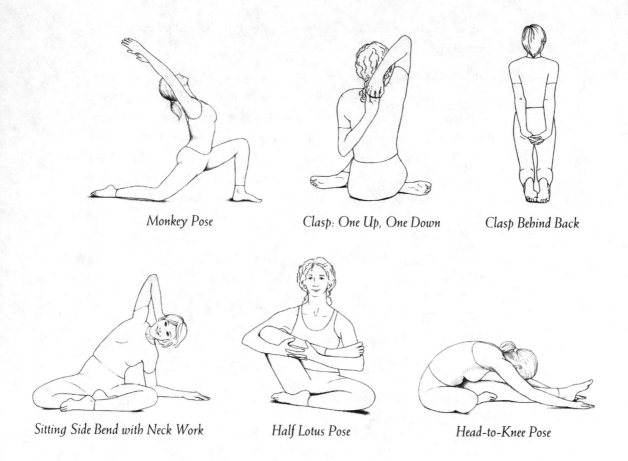

Monkey Pose   Clasp: One Up, One Down   Clasp Behind Back

Sitting Side Bend with Neck Work   Half Lotus Pose   Head-to-Knee Pose

   5. Clasp: Behind Back

   6. Table Top Pose (*Catuspada Pitham*) (pose not pictured; see page 83)

   7. Sitting Side Bend with Neck Work (*Parshvottanasana*)

   8. Half Lotus Pose (*Ardha Padmasana*) or Bound Angle Pose (*Baddha Konasana*)

   9. Head-to-Knee Pose—Forward (*Janu Shirshasana*) or Posterior Stretch
      Pose (*Paschimottanasana*)

  10. Spread Leg Pose (*Upavishtha Konasana*)

  11. Half Spinal Twist Pose (*Ardha Matsyendrasana*)

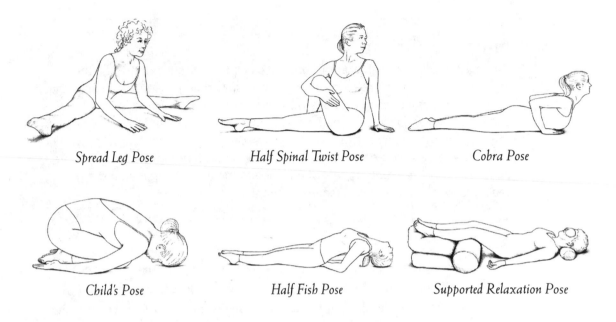

Spread Leg Pose   Half Spinal Twist Pose   Cobra Pose

Child's Pose   Half Fish Pose   Supported Relaxation Pose

12. Cobra Pose (*Bhujangasana*)

13. Child's Pose (*Balasana*)

14. Twist to Flapping Fish Posture Loop (*Shava Udarakarshanasana* to *Matsya Kridasana Vinyasa Krama*) (pose not pictured; see page 81)

15. Abdominal Stretch Pose (*Jathara Parivritta*) or Serpent Side Bend Series (*Anantasana*) (pose not pictured; see page 74 or 75)

16. Half Fish Pose (*Ardha Matsyasana*)

17. Basic Relaxation Pose (*Shavasana*) or Supported Relaxation Pose: Legs on Chair, Feet up Wall, or the Perfect Wedge

Nourishment and cleansing are as important to joint health as to any other part of your body. Perhaps the effects of lack of nourishment and toxicity are not so visibly obvious in the joints as they are in the skin.

SIMPLE SKIN CARE

The skin reacts to changes in all of our tissues, so that whatever imbalances we've been living appear on our skin. Pratima Raichur, director of the Tej Ayurvedic

shape shifting

When attempting to reshape your body, it's helpful to focus not only on the feeling of stretch in the muscles but also on the surrounding tissue. One tissue that is slow to move but can be affected by yoga postures over time is the connective tissue called fascia. As you hold postures regularly, over time you'll be able to gently reshape this slippery wax-like tissue. Focus on its feel when you're in a pose. See if you can locate a sense of something lightly sliding as you stretch. It's not the rubbery feel of muscle stretching but a lighter, more gliding feeling of the muscle's encasement stretching.

Skin Care Clinic, believes our imbalances and life stresses not only can be seen in the skin but show up as accelerated aging in other parts of our body.

The skin develops from the same tissue as the nervous system. Is it any wonder that it reacts with such sensitivity to emotions and stress? Modulation in glandular and nervous system activity that adversely affects the skin can be regulated to some degree through yoga practice. Janice's story illustrates this claim.

After coming to yoga class for about a year, Janice asked if there was anything she could do for her complexion, which was constantly breaking out. Her diet was good, her work was stressful. She drank tons of water. As I considered other factors, I gave her two practices to start off with. I included three rounds of *Kapalabhati Pranayama* with the shoulder stand, both to do daily along with a warm-up practice and a relaxation or whatever other postures she usually did. (She was already remaining in the shoulder stand for ten minutes in class.) I thought this would just be a beginning point for us, and that after I examined other factors in her life and diet, we would make additions. But she didn't contact me again throughout the summer, and I only saw her at a distance in class. A few months later, she came up to thank me. Up close, I was elated to see that her complexion was crystal clear. She was actually sparkling. She reported that to her knowledge, the only difference in her life was those two practices. And she did them every single day!

Along with the lungs, colon, bladder, and the lymph system, the skin is an organ of elimination. Our body is set up to take what it needs and get rid of everything else as waste. If any of these main routes of waste removal are clogged, the body reroutes waste through other channels. Sometimes the skin can't take this much load. There are many well-documented results of people with serious skin problems who were completely cured through fasting and digestive system cleansing. Regular yoga practice supports our body's ability to cleanse through breathing and sweat, and through movements that stimulate and gently manipulate eliminatory organs. Postures like the shoulder stand support the drainage of lymph to its main ports of elimination.

Another thing you can do that is simple and feels great is to dry-brush your skin with a natural fiber brush or cloth made out of hemp. Before you shower, just brush a few strokes everywhere, being careful around your nipples. Use more delicate bristles or just a coarse cloth for your face. This brings circulation to the skin, tones it, and helps it slough off dead cells.

The skin offers protection. As a living interface, it "drinks" what we put on it. Chemicals in deodorants, moisturizers, cosmetics, and even (some believe) in synthetic fabrics are absorbed into our bodies through the skin. This is why it's wise not to put anything on your skin you wouldn't want to eat! So what can we use to moisturize, nourish, and cleanse our skin when it dries out as we get older? For thousands of years, people have used natural oils, legume and grain flours, clay, and salt for skin care.

If your skin is dry, oil it once or twice a day, or as needed, with natural cold-pressed oil. (If your skin is oily, once or twice a week is better.) Buy a few small bottles of oil and experiment; try sesame, sunflower, almond, olive, mustard seed, or coconut. Mustard seed and sesame oils are warming and good in the winter, and coconut and olive oil are cooling and good in the summer. Sesame oil has a lot of nutrients but leaves you smelling a little like popcorn. Almond oil has a sweeter smell. You can, of course, add fragrant essential oils. If you have time, heat the oil by submerging it in hot water or running hot water over the bottle. If you use heavier oils, such as olive or sesame, they may ruin your clothes, so wear an old sweat suit or robe. Then rinse with warm water before you dress. Coconut oil, on the other hand, disappears more easily into the skin.

You can cleanse your facial skin without drying it or subjecting it to harsh chemicals by using natural substances like cream, lemon juice, avocados, bananas, and strawberries. You don't need an expensive salon. Make your own cleansing solution. Combinations of honey and oatmeal or honey and strawberries offer exfoliation and deep cleansing. A banana, milk, and honey mixture is soothing, and banana and avocado can be very restorative.

For the entire body, mix grain or legume flour with oil to form a paste. This is like making a pack (*ubtan*) for your whole body. You can buy wheat, chickpeas, lentils, millet, oats, or barley at health food or Indian grocery stores, or grind the grains yourself if you have an electric grinder. To counteract dryness, add sesame oil in proportion of about two parts flour to one part oil. (If your skin is oily, use water; if it's sensitive, use milk.) I spread an old beach towel on the bathroom floor for this. If the room is warm and you have time, bring something to read and let the pack dry. To keep the drain from clogging, brush the pack off first, then rinse your body with warm water.

Other natural aids to healthy toned skin are exposing it in moderation to air, sunlight, and clean water, all of which contain *prana*.

WEIGHT MANAGEMENT: A LOVING APPROACH TO SOUL CARE

A yogic lifestyle can be of great help in weight management. This is not only because yoga practice can include a fat-mobilizing fitness routine, but because yoga offers us guidance in meeting our needs in a way that agrees with our unique nature and with nature as a whole. Holistic practices such as those offered by yoga address every part of you and your life, so you won't just see dietary suggestions or pointers on exercise. *You* are what this is about, not whatever you think about your weight or your body. Yoga supports you and what you need, and through it you can explore your habits of eating and exercise, time management, and self-care. This is not to judge whether your habits are good or bad, but to gain the necessary insight to transform these habits into ones that serve you better.

Being overweight is the result of a complex number of factors that must be adequately addressed for you to succeed with permanent weight management. Studying your habits and their emotional roots is a long-term commitment to self-understanding that leads to freedom from the yo-yo diet prison. Although weight-loss products are in vast supply, yoga's point of view holds that you cannot separate a weight problem from whatever else you are dealing with in your life.

Being overweight is mostly caused by habits conditioned over time, even though at times hormonal changes have an effect. Cultural roots have an enormous power in determining how we relate to food. Familial eating patterns, learned in infancy and childhood, connect deeply to our emotions and manner in which we accept nurturance. These patterns, set in motion long ago, are usually unconscious. Eating together is belonging. Food is a medium of social behavior, and rejection of it is like rejecting the one offering it. It takes enormous resolve to change course, but change is not just a matter of willpower—it also involves self-acceptance.

Eating is pleasurable; food is sweet. Nature set it up that way so we would survive. Because food is so essential, so delicious, and so much a part of our experience of nourishment, love, comfort, and security, it serves as a perfect substance for fulfillment for our unmet needs. Experts agree that we use food for a variety of emotional purposes, such as reducing stress and anxiety, getting wired for meeting challenges (just go to any Starbuck's before 9:00 A.M.), alleviating depression or boredom, or altering other moods.

Therefore, addressing being overweight requires that we see our habits—whether of cultural, familial, or personal origin—for what they are and work gently with ourselves in constructing a lifestyle that meets our needs in health promoting ways. It's a good idea to seek support in this process.

The basic equation of calories in and calories out is complicated by our body's ancient, and very unconscious, skill in maintaining itself just as it is. Your weight has a set point, controlled by your hypothalamus, that works just like your heater's thermostat. Your body conserves food energy that is not immediately used as fat, so in case you run into a stretch of deprivation, your fat will ensure your survival. Remember, this is ancient programming from the time when people were catching things to eat, not going to drive-thrus. The body is always preparing for this period of famine by storing fat. This is why it's not effective to diet without exercise. When you diet, your body will simply drop its set point to lower your metabolism, burning fuel more slowly to conserve energy, because you've clearly entered a time of scarcity. And because you're not using your muscles much, the body will burn them and other tissues first, so you'll actually end up having lessened your ability to burn fat. Worse yet, when you come off the diet, your body will get busy storing up more fat for when this happens again! It's a nasty cycle.

It's been found that very few people (about 20 percent) who do not exercise are able to keep weight off for more than one year. Lasting weight loss results when the body's set point is lowered. What lowers it? Regular moderate exercise. A threefold approach, including self-study to address detrimental habits, regular moderate exercise, and healthy food habits, is a safe and effective way to manage weight.

Healthful food habits are ones you can live with, not time-consuming, bizarre diet plans for people who don't have lives. They are not so much about what you eat as how you eat. I once worked with a woman, Linda, who lost weight by simply making herself sit down to eat. She is a nurse and a mother who is always caring for someone else. When she gained weight due to a job change that reduced the amount of walking she did at work, she realized her eating habits had gotten out of hand. She cut out the "grab and goes" at the nurse's station and firmly informed her family that when she sat for a meal, they had to fend for themselves. I suggest this method for all mothers who eat their dinner walking somewhere between the table and the stove.

Here are some essential healthful food habits I have gleaned from yogis, yoginis, Ayurvedic physicians, and yoginis who are Ayurvedic physicians. See which ones speak to you, and implement them in your life over time as you can. As Linda proved, they work!

❋ Eat when you're hungry and don't eat when you're not. Keep it in mind and gradually retrain yourself. Becoming aware of what you're doing is the important first step! Use the internal cue of hunger recognition over external ones like mealtime or the sight or smell of food.

❋ When you feel up to it, reduce your portion size by only 10 percent. This will not create a feeling of deprivation, yet you will gradually shrink the size of your stomach.

❋ Slow down! Can you relax for just a moment before eating, and sit for a moment afterward? New moms may have to wait a few years for this.

❋ Pay attention to the act of eating. Many people find it helpful to record in a journal everything they eat.

❋ Chew! Some say thirty-two times per bite. This releases flavor and gives satisfaction. It also takes longer. "Drink your solids and chew your liquids." People who gobble usually gobble more.

❋ Eat at the same time each day whenever possible.

✳ Eat early at night, having the last meal three to four hours before sleep.

✳ Eat in a pleasant atmosphere and not when you're upset.

✳ Always sit down to eat.

✳ Stop when you're less than full. Yogis often say one-third should be food, one-third liquid, and one-third air.

managing hunger

Here are some suggestions for managing hunger, which has to do with that set point mechanism and with not building up such an intense desire for food that you blow all your efforts in one act of satiation.

- Drink herbals teas with honey between meals. Honey has a slight fat-reducing quality. Or try hot water with honey, lemon, and a pinch of pepper.
- Drink water, about two to three quarts each day, depending on your activity level, salt intake, and climate. (This is good for your skin, too!)
- Enjoy sweetness in other aspects of life, such as by watching the sun set, going for a pleasant walk, listening to music, or spending time with family and friends.
- Avoid visually stimulating food settings, such as the Christmas party buffet table or that huge cranberry muffin poster in the subway exit. Go the other way.
- Have a variety of flavors at mealtime: salty, sweet, sour, hot, and so on. This will give you more satisfaction and less craving for more.
- Take supplements so your body will not be deprived of any essential nutrients that could direct you toward a binge.
- When you eat, eat whole natural foods from all the food groups. This will be more energizing and satisfying than if you eat highly processed foods or cut things out.
- Substitute. If you feel you can't resist, eat something that is healthful— such as popcorn, dried fruit, or an apple—rather than something that's unhealthful. Chew sugarless gum. Okay, sugarless gum isn't ancient stuff (though I've heard they used beeswax), but it does help manage hunger.

A MULTIFACETED YOGIC APPROACH TO WEIGHT MANAGEMENT

Swadhyaya. You need to do some self-research to learn about the habits that cause you to overeat or use food in ways that keep weight on. You may also want some help with this. Find a time when you won't be disturbed. Do a brief relaxation. Resolve to witness openly and not judge yourself harshly. This is very important! You may want to draw, move, or write in a journal.

What was a family meal like while you were growing up? What feelings does this recollection evoke? In different sessions, go through your life and reflect on how you related to food and your body at different stages of your development. What was the feeling tone, and how did you feel at these times? What parts were then outside of your awareness? What issues were involved? What events formed habits that you have today? What new information, if any, do you need?

This is a process, which takes time. You may find that what you uncover has less to do with food and more to do with feelings of self-worth, anger at your lot in life, or some other agenda. Observe and lovingly accept all this information. We can't change the past, but we can do things differently in the present, one step at a time.

Sankalpa. Make a resolution to get to the bottom of whatever detrimental habits you have concerning food, exercise, self-image, or whatever information you have uncovered. Seek help from a professional, find a support group, or attend a seminar or workshop. If you can't afford this, local libraries offer free Internet access, where you can find groups that communicate online. Resolve to make changes gradually and in a self-accepting way. Never give up.

Relaxation. Many people eat to gain gratification they are too busy or unable to gain by other means. Often we need time to ourselves, a break or some rest, but we mistake the need for recuperation and a bit of pleasure for the need for food energy. Tension also prevents enjoyment, even during a meal. If you're tense, chances are you're not really paying attention to the act of eating and then aren't deeply satisfied by the flavors and textures of your food. Mothers with small children report they don't even remember eating because mealtime is so filled with distractions. Relaxation, as well as posture practice, develops our ability to attend to internal cues. It helps us figure out just what our needs really are and what will truly satisfy them.

Yoga Practice for Weight Loss

This is a strenuous classical practice that focuses not only on mobilizing fat but also on glandular balance and digestive system stimulation. Feel free to turn any of these practices into a dynamic practice (*vinyasa krama*) or improvisation of breath and movement. Warm up your joints first using the Gentle Joint Limbering Practice.

1. Sun Salutation (*Surya Namaskara*) with Solar Energizer (*Agni Sara*) between repetitions

2. Warrior Dynamic Pose 1 and 2 (*Virabhadrasana Vinyasa Krama* 1 and 2) (poses not pictured; see page 54)

3. Chair Pose (*Utkatasana*)

4. Powerful Pose (*Ugrasana*)

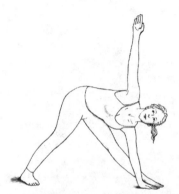

Solar Energizer

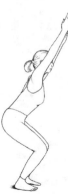

Chair Pose

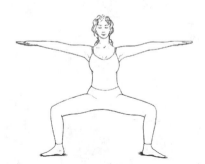

Powerful Pose

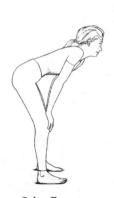

Extended Triangle Pose

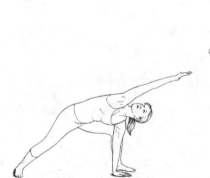

Extended Side Angle Pose

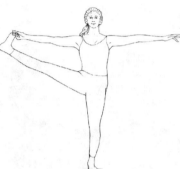

Extended Hand-to-Big Toe Pose—Side

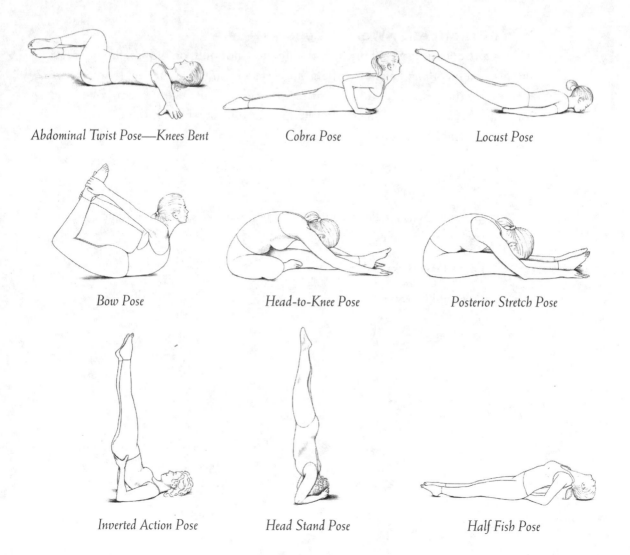

Abdominal Twist Pose—Knees Bent

Cobra Pose

Locust Pose

Bow Pose

Head-to-Knee Pose

Posterior Stretch Pose

Inverted Action Pose

Head Stand Pose

Half Fish Pose

5. Extended Triangle Pose (*Utthita Trikonasana*), Angle Pose (*Konasana*), Revolved Triangle Pose (*Parivritta Trikonasana*) in sequence

6. Extended Side Angle Pose (*Utthita Parshvakonasana*)

7. Side Angle Twist Pose (*Parivritta Parshvakonasana*) (pose not pictured; see page 101)

8. Standing Forward Fold Pose (*Uttanasana*), Big Toe Pose (*Padangusthasana*), or Hand-to-Foot Pose (*Padahastasana*) (poses not shown; see page 110 or 111)

9. Extended Hand-to-Big Toe Pose (*Utthita Hasta Padangusthasana*)—Side or Forward version

10. Upward-Facing Boat Series (*Navasana*) (pose not pictured; see page 45)

11. Abdominal Twist Pose (*Jathara Parivartanasana*)—Knees Bent

12. Double Leg Lift with Solar Energizer (*Utthita Dvipadasana* with *Agni Sara*) (pose not pictured; see page 56)

13. Cobra Pose (*Bhujangasana*)

14. Locust Pose (*Shalabhasana*)

15. Bow Pose (*Dhanurasana*)

16. Head-to-Knee Pose (*Janu Shirshasana*)—Forward and Side versions

17. Posterior Stretch Pose (*Paschimottanasana*)

18. Inverted Action Pose (*Viparita Karani*) or Shoulder Stand Pose (*Sarvangasana*)

19. Head Stand Pose (*Shirshasana*)

20. Half Fish Pose (*Ardha Matsyasana*)

All *pranayama* practices are of benefit, especially *Kapalabhati*.

The habits we have developed throughout our lives are compellingly strong. The ways we satisfy basic needs for recuperation and even contact are of critical importance. When you stifle pacifying habits, the needs they fulfilled remain. Habits by definition operate below our conscious awareness. We may be able to improve our condition through movement and care, but unless we enter into a dialogue with the causes of our habits, it's likely we will follow them again into imbalance. Suggestions for working deeply with yourself through yoga practice are explained in the next part of the book, "Soul Yoga: Look Within."

the fat scraper

An Ayurvedic preparation can support metabolic change so you can reduce fat effectively through diet, exercise, and self-study (*swadhyaya*). The most commonly known compound in the West is Triphala or Triphala Guggulu. You can find it in the supplements section of most large health food stores. (Or see appendix D.) The ingredients are thought to have an *ama*-reducing (fat-scraping) metabolic action.

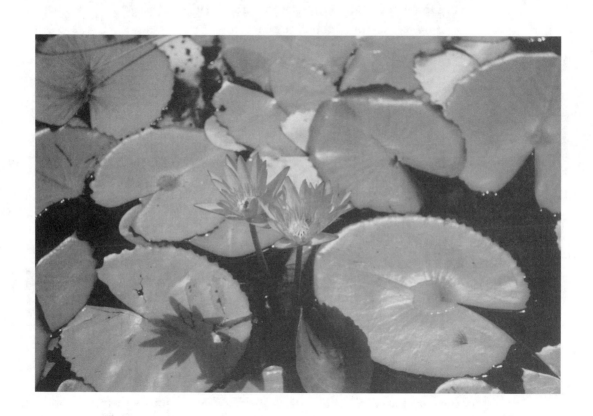

part three

soul yoga:
look within

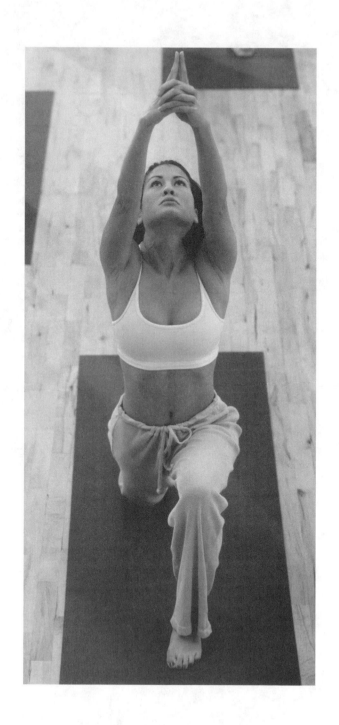

chapter 9

untangle the knots:
inner work using yoga

This being human is a guest-house.
Every moment a new arrival.

A joy, a depression, a meanness,
some momentary awareness comes
as an unexpected visitor.

Welcome and entertain them all!
Even if they're a crowd of sorrows,
who violently sweep your house
empty of its furniture,

Still, treat each guest honorably.
He may be cleaning you out
for some new delight.

The dark thought, the shame, the malice,
meet them at the door laughing,
and invite them in.

Be grateful for whoever comes,
because each has been sent
as a guide from beyond.

—Rumi, "The Guest-House"

Yoga's ability to deliver a reservoir of youth-restoring health and longevity well beyond the norm draws many people to its practice. Those who continue with consistent effort soon learn that vibrant health is only the baseline benefit; they have embarked on a fascinating journey toward wholeness. From a yogic point of view, each soul is like a drop of eternity enlivening the unique swirl of matter that makes up each and every living thing. Thus the soul, or *jiva* in Sanskrit, is both eternal and mortal, perfect and imperfect, at once universal and very personal. Acknowledging this opens us to the paradoxical nature of life. When we limit identity only to what our ego approves of, we cut off the more inclusive, soulful dimensions of our total being that hold tremendous potential.

soul yoga

When you practice yoga systematically, your body becomes resilient, resistant to disease, and strong. The body is the crucible of the soul. Through yoga practice you forge a strong, purified physical container, much like the soft clay of a pot that, once molded and fired in a kiln, can withstand great stress and transport substance. If the body is strong and able to withstand the stress of life, its soul-contents are transformed through practice on and off the yoga mat. If the body is not healthy, it is extremely difficult, if not impossible, to progress on the path leading to yoga's goal of liberation.

As the physical container is fortified, it becomes the medium through which you can address your inner world. Then during practice you can dialogue with deeper recesses of yourself through the nonverbal, nonanalytical medium of the body. The body reveals in its every gesture, movement, and sensation the imaginative life of the soul housed within. When delivered through the body, messages coming from within are powerfully authentic and often surprising! As the body responds to the gentle prodding of the Hatha Yoga postures and movements, vital energy flows through the stuck, closed-off places. When this happens, imagery and feelings come forth into consciousness. It's like opening the door to the attic or to a place where things have been stored for some time. There may be things there you haven't thought of or dealt with in a while.

Since yoga views the ego, or *ahamkara*, as only "the tip of the iceberg" of our total self, it does not devalue any aspect of experience. A signal from the soul can make itself known through any of our perceptual faculties, through an internal sound like a song that springs to mind, or a momentary recollection of a face from long ago. Even a spontaneous movement such as a tic can be an opening to the inner world. As the body dreams, it reveals what your soul, connected to its vastness, would like your ego, established in its individualness, to know. As you work through the meaning of these messages, integrating their significance into your identity, your consciousness expands. With this expansion your personality transforms and develops resilience and endurance, just as the body does through practice.

When we open to the fleeting, synchronistic, odd, or nonsensical messages that come into awareness through the body in practice, we can observe and dialogue with aspects of our physical pain, symptoms, and hang-ups—not to squelch them, but to acknowledge their presence. If we work sensitively enough, we'll receive their messages and integrate their importance into our lives. From this more inclusive perspective, what we ordinarily might consider frightening or problematic contains the key to our salvation. If we honestly follow the thread of meaning back to its source, we uncover its purpose; the tic expresses worry about money, the backache holds anger about a husband's disrespect, the feeling of vulnerability in back-bending poses reveals an unhealed pubescent embarrassment. A signal may express something we have left out and could use more of in our lives. Inner work using yoga gives us concise critical information about what our issues are, what we have denied in ourselves, and which aspects of our personality are up to bat. By working authentically through the body, we arrive at solutions that restore harmony and permit us to follow our life's purpose. Here we are not swallowing whole some vague general guidance from an external source, but cultivating a method of inner guidance that yields solutions perfectly matched to our needs.

Johanna called to tell me about how her yoga inner work led her to make a bold change in her relationship with her boss. Johanna works as a secretary for a middle manager in a large company. As with many secretaries, she knows a lot about the informal power structure of her organization and utilizes this informal network to keep things running smoothly in her department. Here's what she told me:

"I got up to do my sun salutation and noticed my hamstrings were really tight. I thought about what I might have done the day before but couldn't think of anything that would do this to them. I shook them out, massaged them and tried again, but they were really gripping. So I sat down in Posterior Stretch Pose (*Paschimottanasana*) and focused on the tension. I stood up and walked around, exaggerating the feeling of tension in my thighs. It felt like my legs were made of wood."

I asked, "What does this remind me of?"

"The only thing I could think of was that it felt like how I walk around at work. But my legs didn't want to walk; they wanted to stand. Then I saw them as tree trunks sunk into the ground. It was then I realized that I wanted to take a "stand" on some changes that were about to happen at the office, some things that I knew were going to turn out poorly. As a secretary, it's not my place to express my concerns. But I decided to trust my practice, take a chance, and talk with my boss. He was very open to my views, and I think touched by my loyalty and concern. I think he may have shared my ideas with other managers, because I seem to be getting more respect all the way around."

Practice is the safe private place to inquire within and to study one's self and manner of being in the world. In yoga, this self-study is called *swadhyaya*. It also involves studying the teachings of great souls who have traversed the path before us.

Sometimes it's clear what's going on inside us. At other times, we have limited access to knowing what's driving us to act or react the way we do. A strong response to a trifling event may bring up feelings that are hard to place. A mysterious symptom may inadvertently redirect our life course. We can use yoga's methods to get in touch with what's cooking on any given day or at any point in our lives. Through yoga practice we skillfully expand our definition of who we are, enriching our lives by including what at first may seem unincludable.

YOGA'S TWO WINGS

For this pursuit, yoga offers two complementary strategies that work synergistically, like the wings of a bird in flight. They are practice (*abhyasa*) and dispassion (*vairagya*). Both wings are necessary for flight. Practice refers both to the action of doing yoga and to the attentiveness you cultivate as you work with yourself, threading the yoga techniques into all aspects of your life. Dispassion is the attitude of non-attachment, of ever-so-gently lightening your grip on how you want things to go. In this twofold approach, you sort things out, which gives you insight and understanding. At the same time, you step back from involvement with what you observe. This gives you freedom. With these two wings working together, you move forward, overcoming obstacles and heading toward your goal.

SPANDA

In this business of self-discovery, it's essential to remain true to your own initiative and responsiveness. You may have grown up in a situation where relying on your inner guidance system was squelched or denied. Our culture as a whole has ignored the value of intuition and brushed aside the knack women have for tuning in. *Spanda* is a Sanskrit word for spontaneous expression. To me it affirms my right to be alive in this moment exactly as I am, with no shame and no excuses. *Spanda* is often translated as "vibration," but research reveals that the definition of vibration associated with *spanda* concerns that moment of transition from formlessness into manifest form.

A thought is a vibration. You respond to it with some feeling, which creates a symphony of vibratory accompaniment. All this may turn into a physical movement or a series of them that expresses that initial vibratory impulse. Dr. Rudolf Ballentine writes:

> The ancient teachings described *spanda* as a sort of energy of the psyche, a throb or vibration felt by your body that is expressed by your action or, if you haven't acted yet, by your feeling of determination to carry out an action. When you are able to connect with it, you are spontaneous and feel authentic and genuine. . . . This initiates a process of restoring spontaneity, of reforging the natural linkage between what feels right to us and its expression in free and creative activity.

When we allow for spontaneous expression, we move from our own unique dose of vital force. At the time we are open to this authentic energy, we are not caught in duality, but are connected to our power.

following the thread of meaning

Perhaps you have a chronic, nagging physical problem or have pain that can't be diagnosed by a Western doctor. Maybe you're struggling with confusing feelings, or you just haven't had time to stop and digest the events in your life. Yoga practice that is focused on tracking these sensations can help you find meaning in their expression. The images, feelings, and subtle shifts you notice will guide you toward wholeness. Maybe you're entering menopause or have gotten married, divorced, given birth, or lost a loved one. Each life event, for better or worse, requires adjustment, and adjustment means stress. Your practice not only fortifies your health through times of change, but it gives you a way to sort things out and bring parts of your self in from the cold. Then you don't risk stuffing something, hanging onto something, cutting something out, or in other ways not going with the flow of your life. When you process experience physically, you are less likely to stash thought and feeling vibrations that create chemical toxins in your body that are harmful, or act indiscriminately, creating more difficulty in your life. Instead, you develop skill in staying connected to your innermost needs and desires while learning to work effectively with conflict, expectation, and disappointment.

Often the perceptual channels that get less use become the ones that carry messages from within. Because our culture squelches our body's freedom to be expressive and devalues physicality, messages from the soul are often voiced by the body. A signal may arise at any time, not only during yoga practice. It can take practically any form: a symptom, an unintentional tone of voice, an unusual position of the body. Signals like these are easy to spot because they usually seem out of place or a little odd.

CHANNELS OF AWARENESS

Our plan is to depart into inner exploration through movement. We begin with inner sensing of the physical body, called proprioception, in which we pay attention to whatever bodily sensations come into awareness. Then we invite movement, paying attention to our experience as we move. As we work, we may notice information in other perceptual modes. For example, as we move, we might hear an internal sound or become aware of an actual sound in the room. Or our attention might switch to the visual. We might be drawn to some object or color in the room or see an image in our mind's eye as we work. The basic channels of perception are:

❋ Proprioceptive channel (inner physical sensing)

❋ Kinesthetic channel (perception of motion in motion)

❋ Auditory channel (internal or external hearing)

❋ Visual channel (internal or external seeing)

Dr. Arnold Mindell, the creator of Process Work, a Jungian-based method of psychotherapy, describes channels of awareness as avenues through which one is able to track a signal as its meaning unfolds. He also includes more complex channels, such as a relationship channel (our dealings with others) and a world channel (world events that impact us). Mindell analyzed and mapped the way information becomes available as we follow spontaneous expression.

MINING MEANING

Here are some tried-and-true steps to use to follow the meaningful thread of a body signal. This approach to introspection can be considered movement contemplation. You may wish to have someone with you while you work (perhaps taking turns), but this takes you into relationship with that person, so keep that in mind. That person's energy and entire dream field will be present and intermingle with yours. It is in the nature of things.

1. Establish a meta-observer. This is a point of view in which you step back and observe your experience. In meditative traditions, this witnessing stance allows you to detach from your thoughts and emotions so you can watch them dispassionately. When you establish the meta-observer here, it enables you to contain the complexity of whatever comes up by reducing your identification with each part.

2. Tune in. Give yourself a moment for transition. This is especially important if you have been in "doing" mode and have not had a chance to stop and feel your body in a while. Turn your attention inward to proprioception—that is, physical sensory awareness—and do a brief relaxation. First become aware of your breathing; then search your

body from head to toe for patterns of tension. Even at this initial point you may begin to notice information coming into your consciousness on channels of perception other than proprioception. You may see a visual image, such as a gray color to a headache, or hear a sound, perhaps actual ringing in the ears or internal mental chatter.

I did a relaxation prior to writing this section, and when the tension in my back muscles came up, I knew I had a choice. If my goal were to be relaxation, I would focus on the feeling of tension in the muscles and then proceed to soften them. With relaxation practice, I skip perceiving the back tension as a signal of meaningful content and go straight to the task of alleviating it. Straightforward relaxation is a different objective than the one we have here. If I want to delve into the tension as a signal, I focus on it just as it is. So make the tuning-in time brief if you want to mine the body for meaning; otherwise, you may relax away the information available to you.

3. Set yourself up for movement. I attended a workshop presented by a dream analyst. She had us lying on our backs, relaxing and listening to her wonderful voice for quite a long time. Then after some attention to inner imagery, she prodded us to move in response to it. No one stirred! She kept prodding, but no one moved a muscle. How could we? We were way too comfy and flat as pancakes! So set your body up so it will be ready to move. Stand, sit, put your body into a balance pose. Find a starting position that is not too stable. Position yourself as a cube balanced on one corner rather than an Egyptian pyramid as you begin.

4. Select an area of sensation (it could be tension) in your body. Look for the thing that is most odd or unusual, something that seems incongruous with the rest of your experience. As my mentor in this work, Aileen Crow, suggests, "Go for surprise! If you don't, you get something you already know." Focus on the sensation. What information is available? How does it feel? Where is it located? Learn as much as you can about it. Learn so much that your meta-observer could describe it in vivid detail to someone else.

5. Amplify this signal by momentarily encouraging it; feel it more. If it is tension, make it tenser; if it is loud, make it louder, and so on. What-

ever it feels like, see if you can supersize it. As you do this, different things may happen:

- Amplifying the signal may take you into movement. With a little experience, this is usually a good way to go. Allow the movement to happen. If you feel that motion begins but does not continue, go back to your amplification and start again. If this keeps happening, make a loop of it. Start from where the impulse to move begins, go to where it ends, then return to the beginning again. This will produce a rhythmic, repetitive movement loop. You can then amplify this by making the movement loop bigger and by allowing more of your body to participate. Let it move your whole body if you can.
- You perceive additional channel information as you amplify. In the example above of tuning in to my back tension, I chose to amplify it. When I did, I saw in my mind a white racehorse's back muscles. It was straining as it ran, as if it were running at a faster speed than it could sustain for very long. When additional channel information comes through, as in this case, more of the message is filled in. The tension accompanied by the image of the running racehorse gave me a more complete signal to work with.
- You may experience a channel change, taking you completely out of feeling in the body and into some other channel, like the visual channel in the example above. In this case, you become enveloped by the visual information that has come into your awareness. Observe this new information and proceed from there. To follow the trail of signals, amplify each new signal and observe the effect.

Now that you have mined your body for imagery, the question of what to do with it becomes relevant. The answer depends on what came up and what the information is about, but the process of seeing it through remains the same. You merely follow the signal and amplify it as it changes or adds channels. It is truly not possible to know ahead of time what your body will present, just as you don't know when you go to bed what your dreams will be. This practice gives you a chance to immerse yourself in the flow of a single message without being overwhelmed by it. The meta-observer allows you to witness your experience and detach from it.

A signal can be like the awareness of an oncoming weather system. It can be a small squall that turns into a sunny day, or it can begin as a few drops of rain that bring lightning and thunder. Sometimes a signal is just an impression you get that you are in need of something very attainable. Maybe it's just a reminder to slow down. The straining racehorse I saw certainly reminded me that I could not sustain that pace for very long. It can be this simple, and it is wonderful to be able to tune in and listen to such a clear and useful message from the body. As you follow the spontaneous flow of *spanda*, your experience may unfold many things. It may reveal a figure, such as an animal, person, or mythical being come to guide you, or it may unfold two (or more) opposing desires, such as the goal of thinness and the desire to eat sweets. Over time your work may generate a room full of figures that characterize different aspects of your personality.

Things become more complicated when conflict is involved. In this work, you will inevitably come to a point where you reach the limit of your comfort. You no longer want to move according to the signal. Something feels scary, you space out, or you find some excuse for not proceeding. This is quite natural and indicates an internal impasse. You are now at the point of departure into new information about yourself.

This is the time to ask questions. You might ask them of your body, so it can answer through movement, or you might write the questions into your journal and let your thoughts flow spontaneously and unedited onto the page. You might take a blank piece of paper, write a question at the top, and see what you draw in response. Or perhaps you will paint a picture of your experience in this very moment of discomfort, then turn the page and paint from that feeling of discomfort, letting it guide your hand and the brush, all the while tracking your body's responses.

Here are some questions I have found useful in continuing to practice at this juncture:

1. What does this image, feeling, sensation, sound, or situation remind me of? Something from my past? From a dream? From a relationship? From some current life-impression?

2. Who is against expressing this signal? A part of me? A real person or an imaginary one? What is "wrong" with what I'm doing and who is saying it's wrong?

3. If I knew what was about to happen, what would it be?

4. If I knew what parts of me were in conflict, what would they look, sound, and move like? What would each one say? What does each one want? How does each one feel?

5. What does the signal want me to know? What don't I want to know?

As you begin to answer these questions, you will most likely gain information on many channels of awareness at once. Dream images, people in your life, movie stars, magic animals that speak, or figures of mythical stature may arrive—pretty much anything the imagination is capable of is possible here. It is very important that you use your meta-observer to stand back and see what purpose these signals serve by coming into consciousness. Perhaps they will converse with one another. Perhaps they'll fall into a tussle. You may jump into identifying with any of them, but keep your meta-observer as your home base.

You might want someone to witness your work. It's best that they support your meta-observer and not play analyst. You are the one who knows what all this may mean. As Thomas Moore so aptly states in *Care of the Soul*, "There can be no thesaurus of body imagery." This is yet another reason why yoga works. You are ultimately the authority on you. No external expert is going to know better than you do what your signals mean. Yoga practice helps you develop the skills needed to discern for yourself what your signals mean and how they are important in your life. Yoga supports your own inner-guided action. Yes, guidance is available, but if this is truly yoga-based, it will enable you to do your own work.

A GUIDE FOR YOUR GUIDE

Here are some pointers to assist you as you work with yourself in this way.

1. Be patient. You cannot, as it is said, push the river. Paradoxically, an attitude of "doing nothing" will serve you better than an attitude of trying to get to the bottom of something. (Even though you may well be trying to get to the bottom of something!)

2. Because you are entering the imaginative realm, recognize that answers to your questions will not be delivered by Federal Express with

instructions for the rest of your life in a shiny new binder (would it were true!). More likely, you'll be endowed with insight, texture, context, and poetic discourse (sometimes even humor) that will touch you first emotionally, intuitively, and behaviorally. You will receive information and, yes, sometimes instruction, but in the language of art and dream imagery. So tell your rational side that this type of research offers no single tidy sum.

3. Embellish your practice by writing in your journal, drawing, painting, or coming together with other people who are doing inner research as well. For this, yoga centers that value inner processing—such as the Kripalu Center for Yoga and Health, certain meditation groups, and authentic movement groups—are good places to locate others for support.

4. Movement is a hot medium. That is why this work is so powerful, honest, and immediate. When you move spontaneously from *spanda*, it takes you! If you feel frightened or get a jolt of emotion that you don't feel inclined to work with, take the experience out of movement. Change channels. Go visual and shrink the image so you see it on a very tiny screen in your mind. Slow the events way down to slow motion, or make cartoon characters out of the figures and draw them like a cartoon strip. Or do as my daughter suggests: See the monster in its underwear. Such channel changes and controlled additions cool out emotional responses to signals.

5. After working this way alone and with many different people for almost twenty years, I have yet to see the body deliver information the individual personality was not ready for or able to integrate. Resistant to, in denial of, yes, but somehow also ready. But maybe you're not up to the task at the moment the information arrives. Just remember, you can always stop the work! Drop it and do something mundane such as cook, fold laundry, or write thank-you cards. If you want to continue to tackle what has come up, have someone you trust and who knows what you're intention is with you while you work, or seek out a counselor who works from a body-oriented perspective.

This way of working untangles the knots, giving you insight into the deep beliefs, myths, and cultural scripts that can unconsciously direct your life. It is a contemplative practice that involves the body, and so is much more vibrant and immediate than working contemplatively with only the slippery trickster of the mind. A different approach of merit is to develop the point of view of dispassion through sitting meditative practice.

establishing baseline tranquility

Meditation is an effortless focus of attention and awareness. It is different from contemplation, movement or otherwise. In contemplation you take the excursion into the thought or signal that presents itself. In meditation you don't. Instead, you keep the mind focused attentively on the object of your practice, whether that is the breath, an internal sound like a mantra, or a predetermined visual image. When the mind wanders or the body distracts, you simply return to the task at hand, focusing the mind on the meditative object. There are a variety of meditative methods, but all share the aim of bringing you to a point of inner concentration and serenity. Meditation allows you to gradually transfer your identification from projections of the mind to the meta-observer point of view. Over time you find yourself less ensnared by your thoughts and embroiled in your emotions. You develop a calm center that holds your experiences, good and bad, allowing you to see behind the curtain and develop powers of discrimination and accurate insight. In a roundabout way, meditation makes you a more effective person in the world.

PREPARING TO SIT

The actual technique of meditation is simple. However, preparation is the key here, just as in Hatha Yoga practice. Finding a quiet spot at a peaceful time of day is important. To promote consistency, see if you can practice at the same time each day. Freshen up by washing your face and hands, or bathe if this fits into your schedule. Do a few yoga postures to prepare your body for sitting. Breathing and relaxation further prepare your body and mind and, though often overlooked, will take you further in the long run.

In Basic Relaxation Pose (*Shavasana*), Crocodile Pose (*Makarasana*), or Simple Sitting Pose (*Sukhasana*), establish optimal diaphragmatic breathing by bringing your awareness to the cycle of your breath. Allow the breath cycle to become even, so that the inhalation takes roughly the same amount of time as the exhalation. Allow the breath to smooth out by eliminating any jerkiness or changes in tempo. As your body remains in the pose you have chosen, it will cool off and settle. Because of this, you will be able to deepen your breath, extending the time it takes to make one cycle. Do not strain or force. If this is difficult, be sure to include *pranayama* practices in your Hatha Yoga routine.

Once you have established even diaphragmatic breathing, systematically relax your body from head to toes. Relax your head and face. Then relax the neck, then the root of the neck as it goes into the torso. Focus on releasing the arms and hands, then the upper torso, the lower torso, and the legs and feet. All this should take about ten minutes. As this becomes more familiar, you can reduce the time. But if you've got time, I can think of no better gift to give yourself.

Now sit in a way that aligns your head, neck, and torso. Simple Sitting Pose (*Sukhasana*) is a good beginning meditative pose. You may also sit in a chair. Just make sure your feet comfortably reach the floor (use a cushion or book under them if you are vertically challenged).

MEDITATIVE PRACTICE

While there are various possible focal points for meditative practice, we'll use a sound that coordinates with the breath in a specific way. As you inhale, internally hear the sound "so." As you exhale, internally hear the sound "hum." You don't need to say anything out loud; you simply think the sound, hearing it internally on your auditory channel. This object for focus is not religious; it is a pure technique that mimics the sound the body makes when you breathe. It has the effect of quieting and focusing the mind. You may sit for as long as you like or set a period of time for your practice. When ready to end the practice, gently cup your hands over the eyes. Open your eyes, seeing the palms first. Then as you move your hands away, visually reconnect to the external world.

When you meditate, you're going for relaxed, focused attention. Forcing yourself to stay seated longer than is bearable is not recommended. Some days you can sit attentively for long periods with few distractions; other days, whirlwinds of thoughts and emotions blow through in a matter of minutes. Meditation is not about emptying the mind (which is not possible); it's about focusing it. A skill like any other, meditation requires consistent practice. As in your Hatha Yoga practice, how you spend the rest of your day, what thoughts and feelings you attend to, and what decisions you make in your actions all factor into the residue you experience when you sit for meditation. Meditation is a subtle internal practice, so you may wonder whether you're making any progress. If after the first few months you notice you're less reactive, that a quieter state of equanimity begins to prevail, then you're indeed progressing; no histrionics are necessary.

Following the thread of meaning permits you to root out thoughts, beliefs, and habits that cause difficulty for you. Establishing a baseline of tranquility gives you the mental clarity to decisively and dispassionately redirect your efforts in this life. How you choose to employ these practices will depend on what is happening in your life and what your needs are. Yoga is vast, and its methods are varied; you can definitely keep a practice going throughout your entire life if you select and modify what works for you as you grow and change. We all start out looking and feeling great, bursting with the enthusiasm of youth. As we surrender many things to time and age, we recognize the changeable nature of life. Yoga practice helps us enter these changes wittingly. As Pema Chödrön writes, "Only to the extent that we expose ourselves over and over to annihilation can that which is indestructible in us be found." Chapter 10 shows you the range of possibilities for creating a meaningful practice that is personally suited to your needs.

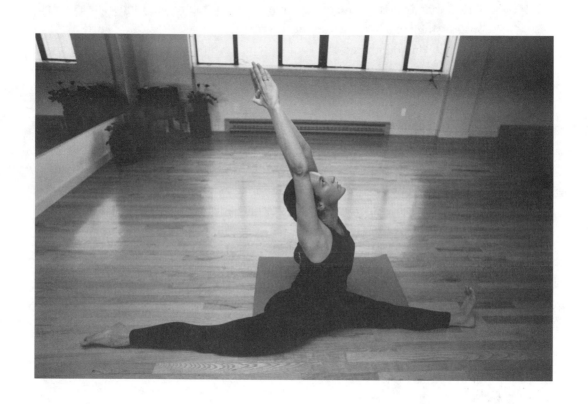

doing it, being it:
the range of yoga practice

The secret of a soul-based life is to allow someone or something other than the usual self to be in charge.
—Thomas Moore

Wisdom comes from peculiarity, not some conformity.
—James Hillman

Nature blesses us with three exceptional gifts for learning: desire to have our needs met, curiosity about the world around us, and a complex nervous system through which we steadily refine our methods for satisfying both these powerful drives. How well we fare through our formative period of early development depends to a large extent on whether or not we are free to explore through movement in a safe and responsive environment. If you have spent any time with children under the age of five, you know they learn by following their curiosity through play, exploration, and experimentation. Putting them into highly structured settings with specific goals usually ends up in frustration for everyone. Through exploration, a child is turned on to learning and moving, and moving to learn more! Delight at unexpected accomplishment, surprise, and fun characterize nature's allure to develop in a balanced and satisfying way.

Most physical culture in the West is goal-oriented. Sign up for ten sessions with a personal trainer, tell her your goals—lose saddlebags, tone up—and you get a list of things you must endure to achieve them. At the gym I see many women who are there to attain goals. They don't enjoy their workout, but are invested in the outcome.

Another approach to physicality harkens back to our playful exploration of youth. Rather than being result-oriented, it is process-oriented. There is an ancient story of renewal told by Clarissa Pinkola Estes called *The Three Gold Hairs*. It tells of a feeble, nearly dead old man, completely worn out, collapsing through the door of an old woman's cottage. The unsurprised woman carries him to the hearth, holds him in her lap, and soothes and rocks him through the night. As she does so, he becomes young again.

Sometimes we don't need a new fitness routine, and we don't need any more challenges! What we need is to slow down and tune in, and in doing so, restore our vital energies. Of several instructions in this story, one is that rest and recuperation are an absolutely necessary and natural part of any endeavor. Slowing down and tuning in doesn't always mean we sleep for days (although this may be what is needed). It may mean we give ourselves the time and space to get clear. We may need to change our perspective, renew our energies, get to the root of something bugging us, or just drop down through a trouble spot that in turn unleashes enormous creative energy.

There are as many approaches to Hatha Yoga practice as there are people in the world. The word *yoga* means union of the individual self with the universal Self. All approaches to yoga share this common aim. I want to encourage you to cultivate your own personal approach, discover your unique personal relationship with yoga's traditional postures and practices. To help you find your way, I have distilled approaches to practice and placed them on a continuum from goal-oriented outer-directed practice to more process-oriented inner-directed practice. A continuum is a spectrum of variations that blend from one extreme to the other. The amount of leeway taken to explore one's inner impulses and responses to the yoga practices is the theme of the continuum described below.

On one end, practices are put onto the body; they are learned and then applied with attention to getting them right by attending to their formal features. In other words, you try to do the yoga practice as perfectly as possible, like a gymnast might attempt to execute a perfect back flip or a dancer would try to perfect a spinning leap in the air. This is the goal-oriented side. On the opposite end, the formal features of the practice are absent. And, although you may have a mission in mind, it takes a back seat to attending to your body's sensations during practice. What you do physically on this far end of the continuum is not planned ahead of time. With this freedom, your practice centers on observing the impulses that emerge from within and are expressed through the body in each moment. You play out an impulse by following its energy, *spanda*, as it emerges into physical movement.

Your yoga practice session is a safe, focused time in which to work with body and soul. Through yoga practice you deepen awareness of subtleties, cultivate powers of observation, and sharpen discrimination. Use these skills as you perform a set routine, or permit your soul to guide your body into movements and positions that reveal meaning. The insights you glean from practice result in changes that propel you along a path of realization of the larger Self within.

the continuum of practice in five stages

A continuum is a blend, but to give examples of how a practice can be done, five distinct approaches are described. They run the gamut from formal to formless practice. Between the two opposite ends of the spectrum, three approaches are described that intertwine these polarities in differing proportions.

STAGE 1. PERFECTION: FOCUS ON THE FORM

This approach focuses on the correct performance of the poses. What you do in the session comes from the outside. You concentrate on getting it right by conforming your body as best you can to the demands of each pose. The goal is to perfect the pose and is similar to the acquisition of athletic skill or artistry in dance. The soul finds value in merging into the archetypal experience of the ancient Hatha Yoga forms. Just as the dancer becomes the dance, the yogi becomes the living embodiment of the pose.

When you practice this way, remain keenly aware of what you're doing. Focus on the exactness of your form and on your breath. Pay attention to your body's sensations to learn how far into the pose to go. Some styles of Hatha Yoga ask you to hold a pose for a certain number of breaths. Even here, be attentive to your body's feedback to decide whether you will or will not hold for the number of breaths suggested. Stay in charge! Even at this more formal end of the continuum, never blindly follow directions, but attend to the body's feedback. Among other benefits, this approach develops mental discrimination. You must stay on top of your reactions in order to mediate between pushing your body too hard and not challenging yourself enough to progress. Discrimination is a valuable life skill that translates readily from the practice session into daily life.

Exercise 1

1. From hands and knees, inhale and push back and up into Downward-Facing Dog Pose (*Adho Mukha Shvanasana*). This posture is described in chapter 3.

2. Focus your attention on perfecting the details of the form of this posture. This includes:

   - Checking to ensure that the creases of the elbows face one another
   - Pressing the knuckles of the hands and toes firmly into the floor
   - Lifting the bones of the buttocks
   - Reaching the heels toward the floor
   - Lengthening the spine
   - Releasing the crown of the head toward the floor

3. Keep the breath even and full, even as you attend to each aspect of the pose.

4. Focus on steadily maintaining the detailed position of this posture while at the same time being mindful of your body's capacity.

5. Release from the pose. Notice the overall effect.

STAGE 2. COMPARISON: THE FORM WITH INSIGHT

This approach also focuses on correctly performing the yoga poses, but leaves some room for introspection. Think of the postures as perfect forms, psychophysical ideals leading to archetypal experiences. When you perform the poses, you are comparing yourself to those ideals. By holding a yoga form, you gain a sense of how well at that moment you embody that form's qualities. In this approach you look at the contrast. You observe your own limitations in assuming the ideal form of the pose. What stands out is your body's unique patterns of tension, strength, tone, and weakness.

Remaining impartial to what we observe can be tricky. The saying "Fools rush in where angels fear to tread" applies because we may have formed habits around comparisons. For example, we may have a habit of measuring ourselves against ideals to see how we fall short and then criticizing ourselves accordingly. Doing this undermines willpower and reinforces the useless pattern of self-criticism. Alternatively, we can choose to observe the habit without investing in it. Not identifying with the motive for a habitual action can be a powerful way to gradually release from it.

By studying our body's limitations, we learn about how we inhabit our own body and lives. Opening to these impressions, we gain insight into how we move through life—arched and open, fearful, compressed, vulnerable, challenging, gripping, powerful, armored, grounded, wishy-washy. These words may describe what we feel as we compare our body's accomplishment of the pose with its ideal form.

Exercise 2

1. Position yourself in Hero Pose (*Virasana*) as described in chapter 4. Find the rhythm of your breathing inside the pose and take time to adjust your posture so it is as correct as you can make it just now.

2. Take a moment to feel yourself in the sculptural form of the pose. Note the demands it places on your body, breath, and mind.

3. Pay attention to where you may be "imperfect" in matching this form. Are you gripping your toes into the floor? Are the shoulders hunched up to the ears? Where do you notice discrepancies?

4. Remain in the pose (or release from it if you feel it is becoming too strenuous). What do you feel? What does this pose bring up in you? Do you feel shy, as if it is asking you to come out of yourself more than your identity allows, or is this stance familiar, even comfortable? Are you doing anything to avoid paying attention to your sensations? What does it feel like to be *you* doing this pose?

5. Note any visual images, internal dialogue, sensations, emotions, or vague states of mind as you attend to the body's sensations. Is anything that came up new?

Being in the posture, breathing, and relaxing with an attentive mind will gently alter your body's resistance and thus your entire state of being.

STAGE 3. VARIATION: DIALOGUING WITH THE FORM

This next approach moves us another step away from formal instruction and toward investigating your body's feedback. With this blend of inner and outer direction, we begin to follow the body's signals as we perform a pose. Here we no longer simply acknowledge or note information, but look for insight into the patterns we use in our lives.

Let's say I'm sitting with my left leg folded in, foot against my inner thigh. My right leg is extended to the front, and I'm reaching forward over it in Head-to-Knee Pose (*Janu Shirshasana*). I've learned that I should keep my extended right knee facing upward in this pose, but it rolls out to the side. In stage 1, the first approach described in this chapter, I would correct this tendency. In the second approach, I would notice this difference, correct it, and notice my response to the correction.

In this third approach, I'm using the posture as if it were a musical theme from which I can depart and to which I can return again and again. I allow my body to lead me into variations. I begin by noticing how my body responds to the requirements of the pose. From here on, I have choices. I may allow my body to do the pose with this personal variation of rolling the leg out to the side. I'm not doing this to cheat the pose by making it more bearable. I'm not sneaking out of stretching my hamstring. I'm giving my body permission to be where it is, for whatever reason, while at the same time being mindful of the "correct" form of the pose. I may move into the correct position if I can and then move back to the rolled-out one, moving back and forth several times. I may experiment with rolling my leg inward to see what this feels like. The variations come from attention to my body's feedback in the moment and not from a yoga book. All the while, I'm tracking my responses. I'm feeling the levels of comfort and discomfort, familiarity and unfamiliarity, and observing my reactions to these sensations.

From here I can make even more choices. I may choose to remain in one of my own variations and attend to the feedback I get from my body. The pose I end up doing may not be the precise one described in a yoga manual, but it is the position that gives me the most useful information; that is, it's right for me. Here I am free to explore the significance of the body's choices as it comes to me through sensation, imagery, or perhaps the mental dialogue I notice as I hold the posture.

Exercise 3

1. Bend forward from your hips into Standing Forward Fold Pose (*Uttanasana*) as described in chapter 3.

2. Take a moment to position your body correctly in the pose and settle into a regular breath rhythm.

3. Remain in this position as long as you like, noticing the effects of the pose.

4. Continue to feel into the body, and as you do, see whether any impulses to alter the pose arise. Is there anything you could change about the pose that would feel just right, give you more information, or make it more interesting?

5. Allow the impetus to lead your body and awareness.

6. If your body elicits no change, you may wish to notice areas not directly affected by the pose, such as your hands and arms. In what ways might they participate? Could you change the position of your legs

to give you slightly different information? Shift your weight into different parts of the feet, step slightly forward, and then to the side with one foot and then the other. Is there something different your head could be doing? Notice where your curiosity takes you. Notice any new impulses to move. Allow this impulse or *spanda* to move your body into new variations of the pose.

STAGE 4. DEPARTURE: THE FORM INTO MOVEMENT

Shifting toward the formless side of the continuum, this approach uses the postures as points of departure to explore the body's signals through movement. The focus now shifts toward following *spanda*, or the inner drive to move. Not yet jumping into the open waters of formlessness, we begin in a formal pose and keep familiar yoga postures in mind so that we'll recognize them if we come upon them in our movement journey. Perhaps we'll return to the beginning pose or the movements will take us to different postures, or perhaps not.

This time, focus on the impetus to move or change positions, and when you give in to this impulse, be mindful of the going. For example, in the Seated Forward Bend (*Janu Shirshasana*), with one leg folded in and the other leg extended, I may again notice my extended leg turning out to the side as I reach forward. Because I am letting go of the form even more now, I may decide to play with this action. I reach forward and my extended leg rolls out. I sit up and the leg rolls in. If I repeat this back and forth movement and coordinate it with my breathing, I've created a personal *vinyasa*, or moving posture loop. It's the result of combining the yoga vocabulary with my own idiosyncratic tensions in the moment.

As I move through the pattern, it may transform into something else. For example, without directing it, I may lift and arch as I sit up, or circle my torso to the side. This occurs not because I think "What shall I do next to make this more interesting?" but because my ego has stopped directing and has allowed my body the freedom to spontaneously move. I now have the opportunity to observe the flow of my responses to this exploration.

Exercise 4

Perform Standing Side Stretch Pose (*Ardha Chandrasana*) as described in chapter 4.

1. Allow the body to settle into the position and the breath to settle into a rhythm. Remain in the pose for as long as you like. Pay attention to the sensations in your body, the effects of the pose. Notice the movement the body is already doing. Notice any impulse to change positions or add to this movement in some large or small way.

2. Allow this impulse or your curiosity to lead your body into movement, even if it seems odd, silly, or purposeless to do so.

3. Continue to allow the body to move freely. You may keep in mind the posture used as the point of departure. Is there another posture this movement is similar to, passes through, or is heading toward? Observe how your body relates to or dances around these forms.

4. Continue to pay attention to the flow of your awareness. What images, feelings, and internal dialogue, if any, accompany this journey?

5. To end, simply allow the body to settle in a position of rest.

Note: If at any point you find you are doing movements that bring up something you are not willing to experience, just stop moving! Turn your attention to some mundane thing. Look out the window. Let this work go for now.

STAGE 5. IMPULSE: MOVEMENT EXPLORATION AS PRACTICE

At this end of the continuum, we begin with no physical forms or formal structure to the practice time. Instead, what is required is suspension of sense-making, release from expectation, and willingness to remain aware of what is happening in the present moment. With no given plan to enact, the body becomes the medium through which inner impulses manifest into tangible forms. Rather than directing the body through some motions, we begin by observing the flow of sensation in the body.

As you observe what's happening in your awareness, you may have an impulse to move. It could be to get more comfortable or to release tension in your neck. It could be to stretch or to collapse. If you're standing, you might begin with an almost imperceptible swaying motion. Or you may find that you remain still and your mind flows without bringing your body into motion.

What happens is entirely open to what presents itself to your awareness in the moment. You simply stay present to what is happening as it transpires and allow your body to move according to the sensations and impulses coming into your awareness.

With this approach, the body is free to move or hold whatever position feels right, even though the analytical mind may not be able to explain why this is so. This may take a little getting used to, especially if you don't often permit your body to lead. You may feel self-conscious at first. Since the medium of movement is fluid and nonverbal, what comes forth is likely to be overlooked by internal critics. Because you may lose track of time, set a time limit for this kind of practice.

The movements you end up doing may come from various levels of your being. The process is a little like mining for gold. You don't know exactly what, if anything, you will find. The gold may be too deeply embedded, or you may strike a vein. Movement coming from a stiff neck could be a simple release from driving in rush-hour traffic. Or it could express a readiness to release a rigid concern for social conformity that has caused you to stiffen up over many years. Another scenario could be that the movement brought on by the sensation of stiffness in your neck turns into an exotic playful dance that reminds you of how much fun it is to be alive. There's no telling beforehand what the signals will mean or where the journey will take you. This is a wondrous mystery, a fantastic trek into the many facets of self and life energy. If you enjoy working this way, over time you may notice themes or patterns emerging that you'll interpret. Or you may never expose these experiences to translation.

Exercise 5

1. Set a time limit for your practice. A kitchen timer or a watch with an alarm is useful. A large clear space is best. Give yourself some additional time to transition out of your practice after working this way.

2. Begin in any position that suits you. However, if you choose a position that is extremely stable, such as lying face down on the floor, it may take you all your practice time to initiate movement.

3. Pay attention to the flow of sensations in the body, to whatever impressions come into your awareness. They may be physical sensations or impulses to move. You may pick up internal dialogue, an emotional

tone, or a visual image. Resist making something up. Just attend to what is happening in this moment.

4. Follow the flow of awareness into whatever happens next. Once again, if something comes into awareness that makes you extremely uncomfortable for whatever reason, just stop.

5. Give your body permission to move in response to what you are experiencing. If you don't wish to follow what is happening in movement, get some blank paper and draw, retaining the quality of motion or the image you saw.

6. Stop whenever you have had enough or when your time is up.

The purpose of this continuum is to give you some ideas about *how* to approach yoga practice so it will fit your needs exactly on any particular day or at any time in your life. Exploring different ways of uniting with yoga will keep your relationship with your yoga practice vital, meaningful, and full of soul. By all means, mix things up.

Here's an example of a practical way to organize your approach to practice. During the week when time is tight, approach practice from the formal side of the spectrum. Learn the poses and match your body to them as best you can. Then on the weekend, when there is more time, work from the formless side. This side is also good when you're troubled with something, sick, or even just plain bored with formal practice. Someone could argue that you're avoiding a learning experience by not meeting boredom head on. This may be true. As long as you observe your own reactions and responses to what you're doing, you'll know if you're copping out or creatively coping. Attentive exploration and experimentation are the keys.

The sky was the color of a gray woolen coat, a dense texture of moisture and smoke from the cooking fire. Standing on spongy clumps of grass near a Himalayan mountain peak, our camp for the night, I asked Swami Veda about an internal conflict I was having. There in India, my meditation practice was blossoming. I noticed immediate changes in my outlook and in the way I was handling stress. Yet prior to coming to India, I had made huge breakthroughs by working attentively with my body in movement. I had retrieved some significant events from my past and saw how they had been unconsciously functioning in my life up until then.

Days from anywhere, with only the sight of mountain peaks fading in the distance and the tinkling sound of bells on horses clomping past, I was losing my grip on my sense of identity, Judeo-Christian upbringing, and worldview. Because yoga had returned to its place at the center of my life, and along with it the gentle redirecting of meditation, I was afraid I would have to deny the importance of using my body's intelligence to work through issues in my life. I felt the self-work I did both in India and America were essentially the same. To me they were both yoga; only the approach was different. Swami Veda listened steadily to my words. I'm certain he took in my earnest sense of struggle as well. I can still see him, fire lighting half his face and beard, as he said: "In the West you focus on getting it right. The correct answer has to be only one thing. But in reality, more than one thing can be the answer. Think in terms of both/and instead of either/or and you will not make problems for yourself."

You may find that some yoga schools adhere strictly to their definition of yoga or to "getting it right," while others smile openly in all directions, acknowledging that "paths are many. Truth is one." The practice of yoga is beyond any specific method or technique, just as the experience of the Divine is beyond any concept or word used to describe it.

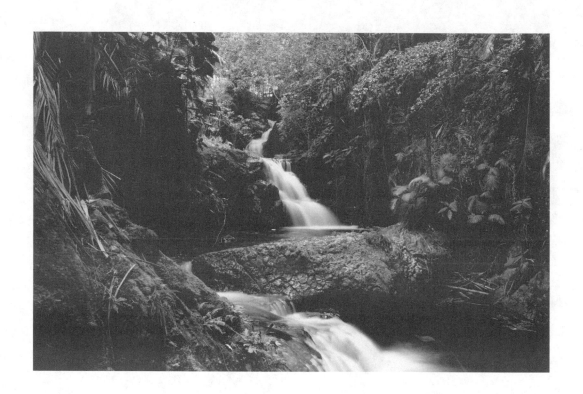

part four

*your own yoga:
a place for practice
in your life*

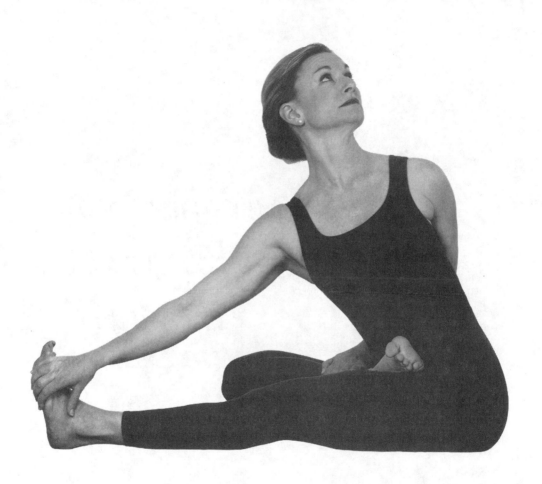

chapter 11

yoga your way:
creating your own practice

We must keep remembering that our bodies respond to the feminine principle. They respond to rest, nurturing, to a presence that says you are OK just the way you are.

—Christiane Northrup

It helps to remember that our practice is not about accomplishing anything—not about winning or losing—but about ceasing to struggle and relaxing as it is.

—Pema Chödrön

What if you had a best friend who never let you down and could give you exactly what was best for you? This friend would anticipate your needs even before you could consciously express them and give you exactly what you need right on time.

Your yoga practice can be like this best friend. It can help you to know what your body and soul yearn for before your conscious mind has an opportunity to explain away these important insights. Designing a practice that suits you like a finely tailored garment is a creative act you can enjoy each day. Adjust your practice by merely following your process, feeling into yourself, and trusting the wisdom that is expressed from within. Yoga works like any other sort of training, but this training is not to help you win a race or play a sonata; it is training to hold on to wholeness and a meaningful, balanced life. A musician learns the scales and chords and studies a variety of different compositions and styles. Yet at some point, she turns the lesson book over and plays from her heart. My aim is to present you with lots of useful options so that yoga can become an adaptable yet reliable support for whatever you need in order to live a meaningful, self-loving life.

designer yoga

Even though it's necessary to leave the door open to possibility, it's equally good to have a flexible plan. One day you may want to work from a blank slate. On another day, a routine you can surf through without soul-searching fits the bill. A practice you can live with is the topic of this chapter. In designing your own program, keep in mind what you want from it. Do you want to reduce anxiety, study your dreams, get in shape, learn your life's purpose, or have better posture at your desk job? You can design and redesign practice programs to match your needs as your life, schedule, health, and interests change. Working with the order in which you do the poses is like choreographing a dance or composing a piece of music. You can play with the phrasing, tempo, and emphasis. As you create, keep in mind that a well-ordered sequence will help you recover from preceding practices and prepare you for what is to come.

The posture chapters present nine categories of yoga poses. If you choose one or more practices from each category, plus *pranayama*, and a beginning and ending transition, you will have a balanced yoga practice. Your beginning transition could be a luxurious relaxation done in the Basic Relaxation Pose (*Shavasana*), or a few breaths standing in the Simple Standing Pose (*Tadasana*). Or you might sit erect in the Simple Sitting Pose (*Sukhasana*) to observe your mind as it comes to rest on your breath. Relax once again at the end of your practice and at any time you feel tired. Take an additional moment at the end for integration if you have time. Record technical notes or meaningful insights in your log or journal. This is also an excellent time for meditation. Integration time is the icing on the cake that reinforces your desire to practice and hastens your progress.

Table 11.1 shows a template for designing a formal practice routine. Use this template as you would a restaurant menu: Choose an appetizer, an entree, two vegetables, and so on. If you choose from each category, you've got a basic balanced yoga practice. You may do the practices either by following the template's outline or organizing them by body position—standing poses first, then sitting, then lying down. As you become familiar with how they feel, arrange them so they offer recuperation—that is, if you bend back, bend forward; if you cross, open; if you're upside down for awhile, recuperate right side up. The possibilities are truly limitless.

Look through the book and select what interests you. Be creative—it's really fun! Or build a basic practice around posture recommendations from the specific sections of chapters 3, 4, and 5. Or, if you prefer, use one of the basic practice routines outlined below as a point of departure. The template has columns for notes of different kinds. For example, one client modified this template to address neck pain. Her goals and comments revolved solely around her neck's response to the practices. If your imagination comes alive via your visual channel, keep a drawing pad handy as you practice or adapt the template to include drawings.

Of course, you may find yourself smack-dab in the middle of the perfect practice sequence and discover a new pain in your back or hip, an emotion such as apprehension, or gratitude that wasn't there before. At this point, your desire to explore signals such as these may mean you drop the plan to follow your interest. Rest assured that sensing inwardly and following your curiosity are very important aspects of yoga practice. You can come back to the plan tomorrow—or alter it, based on what you learn from these signals today.

Table 11.1   Template for Basic Yoga Practice

Date: _____   Practice Time: _____   Practice Goal: _____

ELEMENTS	PRACTICE CHOICES Circle One: *Asana/Vinyasa/* Make It Easier/ Challenge Me	APPROACH Number of Times Repeated Breath Counts in Pose Heating/Cooling Pose/Counterpose
1. Centering		
2. Limbering		
3. Pelvic Center		
4. Whole Body Integration		
5. Balance		
6. Side Bending		
7. Shoulder Mobility and Back Bending		
8. Twisting		
9. Hip Mobility and Forward Bending		
10. Inversions		
11. *Pranayama*		
12. Relaxation		
13. Integration Time		

Table 11.1   *(continued)*

	OBSERVATIONS Insights, Discoveries, Questions	SUGGESTIONS Inspirations Alterations
ELEMENTS		
1. Centering		
2. Limbering		
3. Pelvic Center		
4. Whole Body Integration		
5. Balance		
6. Side Bending		
7. Shoulder Mobility and Back Bending		
8. Twisting		
9. Hip Mobility and Forward Bending		
10. Inversions		
11. *Pranayama*		
12. Relaxation		
13. Integration Time		

off the rack

If you prefer to let me drive, here are three practices from the formal side of the continuum. The first two are basic beginning practices. The third one is more challenging. They are balanced practices with many benefits, so you can use them forever and never have to create one of your own. The first one follows the order of the template. The other two include practices from every category but in a progression different from the template. As you gain confidence and familiarity with these practices, you may decide to make meaningful alterations in these routines over time.

To do a beginning basic practice, perform each pose and each side of each pose one time. Holding a pose for three breaths is a good minimum starting point. Add repetitions and numbers of breaths as your interest and capacity dictate. On the top end, when you can do three repetitions with ten breaths in each pose from the first two practice routines, go on to routine 3. When you can do the same there, you'll need to go on to a more challenging practice to make progress. (See the "Body Beautiful" practices in chapter 8.) With the dynamic poses, you are breathing and moving together. Begin at three repetitions and work up to eight, depending on your capacity. Watch your breathing. If it shortens as you move, you're straining. Reduce the number of repetitions until you can perform each one with a long, even breath cycle. Then gradually add more.

BASIC FORMAL PRACTICE 1

(Use the most comfortable version of the pose from the main description or from the "Make It Easier" or "Challenge Me" variations.)

1. Centering: Centering and Relaxation in Simple Sitting Pose (*Sukhasana*) with attention to diaphragmatic breathing

2. Limbering: Gentle Limbering (from side bar in chapter 3) Sun Salutation (*Surya Namaskara*)—Repeat 2 to 4 times

3. Pelvic Center: Root Lock (*Mula Bandha*)

Abdominal Lift (*Uddiyana Bandha*)

4. Whole Body: Extended Triangle Pose (*Utthita Trikonasana*)

Downward-Facing Dog Pose (*Adho Mukha Shvanasana*)

5. Balance: Tree Pose (*Vrikshasana*)

6. Side Bends: Half Moon Pose (*Ardha Chandrasana*)

Extended Side Angle Pose (*Utthita Parshvakonasana*)

7. Shoulder Mobility: Elbows Cross in Front

Clasp—One Up, One Down

Clasp—Behind Back

Table Top Pose (*Catuspada Pitham*)

Upward-Facing Plank Pose (*Purvottanasana*)

8. Backward Bending: Cobra Pose (*Bhujangasana*)

Half Bow Pose (*Ardha Dhanurasana*) or
Bow Pose (*Dhanurasana*)

9. Twisting: Universal Twist Pose (*Shava Udarakarshanasana*)

10. Hip Mobility   Half Lotus Pose (*Ardha Padmasana*)

11. Forward Bending: Bound Angle Pose (*Baddha Konasana*)

Half Hero Pose (*Ardha Virasana*)

Head-to-Knee Pose (*Janu Shirshasana*)—Forward
or Single-Leg Lift Pose (*Utthita Ekapadasana*)

Child's Pose (*Balasana*)

12. Inverted Poses: Inverted Action Pose (*Viparita Karani*)

Plow Pose (*Halasana*)

Half Fish Pose* (*Ardha Matsyasana*)

13. *Pranayama*:   Alternate Nostril Breathing (*Nadi Shodhanan*)—
9 or more rounds

* Use Half Fish Pose after Inverted Action Pose and Plow Pose if you have been inverted for more than a few minutes.

14. Relaxation: Basic Relaxation Pose (*Shavasana*)—Relax from head to toe and focus on even diaphragmatic breathing for ten minutes

15. Integration Time

BASIC FORMAL PRACTICE 2

Use whichever version of the pose you can do most comfortably.

1. Basic Relaxation Pose (*Shavasana*)

2. Solar Energizer (*Agni Sara*)

3. Sun Salutation (*Surya Namaskara*)—2 to 4 times

4. Warrior Dynamic Pose 1 or 2 (*Virabhadrasana Vinyasa Krama 1, 2*)— Do one or both.

5. Extended Triangle Pose (*Utthita Trikonasana*)

6. Angle Pose (*Konasana*)

7. Revolved Triangle Pose (*Parivritta Trikonasana*)

8. King Dancer Pose (*Natarajasana*)

9. Standing Forward Fold Pose (*Uttanasana*)

10. Crocodile Pose (*Makarasana*)

11. Cobra Pose (*Bhujangasana*)

12. Downward-Facing Boat Pose (*Adho Mukha Navasana*)

13. Child's Pose (*Balasana*)

14. Sitting Twist Pose (*Bharadvajasana*)

15. Bound Angle Pose and/or Reclined Bound Angle Pose (*Baddha Konasana*)

16. Posterior Stretch Pose (*Paschimottanasana*)

17. Sitting Side Bend with Neck Work (*Parshvottanasana*)

18. Head-to-Knee Pose (*Janu Shirshasana*)—Side

19. Half Circle Pose (*Ardha Chandrasana*)

20. Half Upward-Facing Boat Pose (*Ardha Navasana*)—Upper and then Lower

21. Bridge Pose (*Setu Bandhasana*)

22. Inverted Action Pose (*Viparita Karani*)

23. Plow Pose (*Halasana*)

24. Half Fish Pose (*Ardha Matsyasana*)

25. *Pranayama* in Simple Sitting Pose (*Sukhasana*): 2-to-1 Ratioed Breathing

26. *Pranayama* in Simple Sitting Pose (*Sukhasana*): Vocalization

27. *Pranayama* in Basic Relaxation Pose (*Shavasana*): Optimal Diaphragmatic Breathing

MORE CHALLENGING FORMAL PRACTICE 3

1. Simple Standing Pose (*Tadasana*), focus on breathing

2. Gentle Limbering: Sun Salutation (*Surya Namaskara*) with Solar Energizer (*Agni Sara*) done between repetitions—4 to 6 repetitions

3. Chair Pose with Solar Energizer (*Utkatasana* with *Agni Sara*)

4. Powerful Dynamic Pose (*Ugrasana Vinyasana Krama*)

5. Warrior Dynamic Pose 2 (*Virabhadrasana Vinyasa Krama*)

6. Extended Triangle Pose (*Utthita Trikonasana*), Angle Pose (*Konasana*), and Revolved Triangle Pose (*Parivritta Trikonasana*) done in series—3 to 5 repetitions in each position before repeating on other side

7. Extended Hand-to-Big-Toe Pose (*Utthita Hasta Padangusthasana*)—Forward and Side

8. Tree Pose with Forward Fold (*Vrikshasana*)

9. Four-Limb Staff Pose (*Chaturanga Dandasana*)

10. Side Plank Pose (*Vasisthasana*)

11. Camel Pose (*Ushtrasana*)

12. Child's Pose (*Balasana*)

13. Double Leg Lifts (*Utthita Dvipadasana*) with Solar Energizer (*Agni Sara*)

14. Upward-Facing Boat Dynamic Pose 1 or 2 or both (*Navasana Vinyasa Krama* 1, 2)

15. Desk Pose (*Dvipada Pitham*)

16. Bound Angle Pose (*Baddha Konasana*)

17. Posterior Stretch (*Paschimottanasana*)

18. Spread Leg Pose (*Upavishtha Konasana*)

19. Half Spinal Twist Pose (*Ardha Matsyendrasana*) or Spinal Twist Pose (*Matsyendrasana*)

20. Shoulder Stand (*Sarvangasana*)

21. Plow Pose (*Halasana*)

22. Half Fish Pose (*Ardha Matsyasana*) or Fish Pose (*Matsyasana*)

23. Dolphin Pose or Scorpion Pose (*Vrishchikasana*)

24. Head Stand Pose (*Shirshasana*)

25. Simple Standing Pose (*Tadasana*)

26. *Pranayama* in Simple Sitting Pose (*Sukhasana*): Alternate Nostril Breathing (*Nadi Shodhanam*)

27. *Pranayama* in Simple Sitting Pose (*Sukhasana*): Vocalization

28. *Pranayama* in Basic Relaxation Pose (*Shavasana*) or Crocodile Pose (*Makarasana*): Healing *Pranayama*

work your rhythm

Getting a regular practice rolling in your life requires several fundamentals. The practice needs to be ultimately doable—not too long, difficult, or boring. It also needs to take place at a time when you have no food in your stomach, like just before a major meal or a few hours after a smaller one. For most of us, this requirement—in concert with other obligations like work, carpooling children, cooking meals, or toddler naps—whittles down options for practice times considerably. But the most crucial factor in successfully sticking the landing of yoga in your life is commitment. You must schedule your practice as you would a dental appointment for a very bad toothache. At first, plan to practice two or three days a week. Write your practice times down in your date book: "Yoga practice—5:30 to 6:45." Add more as you can. You must ardently defend this time.

Oprah Winfrey has said many times that we teach people how to treat us. Teach anyone who threatens your practice, even your cherubs, that it is of the utmost importance and that you *will* take the time to do it consistently. If you're a generous Good Samaritan who is easily talked into sacrifice and you don't feel up to defending your practice time to coercive others, don't tell them what the time is for! You have an appointment (with your "Self") and you can't miss it. Think of the other activities you plan for and carry out. This is just as important—maybe more so.

That first break in the routine is the hardest. If your family is used to your round-the-clock availability, and all of a sudden your door is closed for an hour and a half, it may feel weird *at first.* One night I called my friend Carolyn. Her son politely told me she was busy. I asserted, "Sure, Mikey, but just tell her it's Jaime." To my amazement, Mikey, who I think was nine at the time, replied, "Mommie is meditating and she won't be available until ten, which is after my bedtime." Communicate. They will adjust. Who knows—they might even join you. Meanwhile, you'll be modeling integrity, self-care, and self-discipline.

Your aim is to build a comfortable habit that fits into your life, one that you'll miss if you don't do it. Our body's attunement with nature provides a few ideal times to practice throughout the day. The first is early morning, preferably before 6:00 A.M.. (Are you laughing?) The second is around noon, before lunch. A practice at this time stokes digestion. The third time is late afternoon between 5:00 and 6:00 P.M., and finally in the evening, finishing by 10:00. (If you practice later and do heating work, you may not be able to fall asleep, because this part of the day is ruled by *pitta* or the fire element.) When I teach, I use humor as a way to acknowledge the difficulty of embedding yoga practice into dizzyingly busy lives.

One time I urged students to practice balance poses in the kitchen while cooking dinner. I suggested they fit the Tree Pose in while chopping vegetables, and perhaps try the Standing Scale Pose, in which you bend over 90 degrees with your back leg out, while searching lower shelves of the refrigerator for errant heads of lettuce. With absolute seriousness, a woman of tender age responded, "But aren't you supposed to practice in silence, alone in a clean and quiet room?" Before I could acknowledge her statement, another class member replied, "Yeah, if you have a clean quiet room."

Brooke was new to our intermediate/advanced class. She heard some of us joking about how dark and cold it is when we get up at 4:30 A.M. to do practice. She decided she would do this, too, but shortly gave up. She reported that she was so tired by the end of her very demanding day that she could barely think straight. So she does an evening practice to wind down. This matches her needs.

Lydia is an attorney and mother of three. She does two days a week of early morning practice before her kids get up. (The other three weekday mornings she walks on her treadmill.) She gets in a fifteen-minute office yoga practice when she can, mostly breathing, upper body stretches, and relaxation at her desk. On Saturday mornings, she takes a yoga class with her teenage daughter while her husband takes the boys to soccer. This is her limit. She fits her practice in so it can support her health and the rhythm of her life. When can you fit it in?

Sometimes the practice is to just make a space for you in your life! You might spend the hour draped over a bolster or with your feet up the wall. You may tap into dream imagery that you had forgotten and write feverishly in your journal during your time. A yoga master of our time, T. K. V. Desikachar, has said that whatever serves the individual is right. Work your rhythm.

keep your practice afloat

When you begin, your practice is like a thin cotton thread. (You struggle to find time to pick it up and make a few stitches.) As the habit of practice forms, the thread gets stronger. Now instead of finding time to try this yoga stuff out, it becomes a strong cord that threads together the different aspects of your life. Each day may be framed by practice. As your practice becomes a well-worn part of your day-to-day existence, its influence increases so that the rest of the day actually seems to fit in around practice! Life events become arenas in which you try out what you learn from your yoga. Yoga means union, and through practice you unite with your Source, so that no matter what happens, you're fortified by inner resources that you contact and cultivate through practice.

Most training programs fail not because of difficulty but due to boredom. Working through plateaus is an important life skill that builds self-confidence and will power. The word in Sanskrit for resolve is *sankalpa*. This is necessary to keep your practice going. The Nike slogan "Just do it" urges us to move from our *sankalpa*. When I trained for my first distance cycling event, I had to learn to ride over mountains. On the steep parts, I was terrified that I would fall over with my feet clipped in and get run over. My cycling mentor, Mark Manczak, would say, "It's just you out there; it's all up to you," and that would scare me even more! Up to me? But my yoga practice taught me how to hold the dynamic pose of pushing up that monstrous hill without giving in to the terror in my pounding heart. Yoga taught me to witness my experience. As if from far away, I saw someone scared nearly to death, alone on that mountainside, and felt a brilliantly burning resolve to keep going that outranked my fear.

A bird in flight is an image commonly used in yogic literature. I have heard the image used to depict the challenge of yoga practice in our lives. The head of the bird represents the willpower and faith (*shraddha*) required to channel life toward one's goal. The tail represents the drag of the endless array of obstacles that impede progress (*mahat*). The wings represent the tools needed to succeed in the face of obstacles. They are yoga practice (*abhyasa*) and dispassion (*vairagya*). We can't control what will happen in our lives, but we can learn to shape our internal world through yoga practice.

Resolve is necessary at the outset, but it must be reinitiated over and over (and over) again. Consistency in practice over time results in yoga's benefits. Hundreds of people have come to me for practice routines, and most of them have that piece of paper stuffed in a drawer somewhere. But this doesn't matter. What matters is that they dig it out once more and begin again. One of the greatest souls alive in our world today, Mata Amritanandamayi, says, "You do not know the progress you are making, so do not give up."

As you practice, pay attention to what fascinates or delights you. Maria is in love with the sense of comfort and serenity she finds in her gentle practice. An architect by profession, she has made such a beautiful practice space in her home that it makes sense she wants to be there on her luxurious futon mat as much as possible. The details of meaning that resonate from within her prompted her to create a space that affords her a soul haven.

I'm not the least concerned with my practice environment, but I am riveted by what I call metaphysical themes that I explore through the different postures. When I come to a particularly boring pose, or one that I squirm through, I take my dullness or resistance as a sign that there may be some unconscious material brought into focus by the pose. When I hit on something like this, I don't force my body to hold or deepen, but sit at the edge of my discomfort and ask a few questions, such as "What created this closing down in the body?" or "Who's against opening in this way?" I might ask questions related to what the pose requires, be it standing tall, balancing, yielding into the ground, or asserting myself by pushing out of it. I might ask, "What is it you wish to express but can't?" or "What are you afraid of?" and "Who can help you?" When I practice this way, I'm not sculpting my muscles like clay or trying to get into a dress size.

When I work this way, my body is my link to nature and the medium of my soul. The deeper concerns that I cannot yet hear as words—such as feelings of grief, rejection, or love that I have not taken time for or have rationalized away—surface here in my body's language of breath and movement. Practicing this way, I am connected to the whole of my life. My story is recreated and reintegrated each day through my body so that my life's purpose and the actions of my days are reunited through yoga.

Metaphysical themes are about any issues that are expressed through your body. Some women have issues about being or appearing strong, so poses like the Warrior Pose are difficult. For others, reaching out in a supported way is not a familiar gesture. The practice, then, is to learn through the body how to reach with internal support. This skill can then be translated into the business of daily living, where saying "No. I cannot extend myself any farther without hurting myself" is the application.

To practice with an awareness of what the body reveals through the poses brings us into a transformative dream space of creative possibility. Practice is no longer a humdrum, by-the-clock occupation. It becomes a powerful adventure of self-discovery and transformation.

Whether you choose to use your practice to stay connected to your inner life or not, here are a few tips to keep your practice going.

1. Plan your practice times. Write them into your engagement book or calendar as you would any other appointment.

2. Set the stage. If your practice space is used for other activities and by other people, set it up for your use before you begin. Nothing can blow it all at the last minute more than walking into a room filled with "stuff" when you yourself need some clearing!

3. Turn off the phone and let everyone know you are not to be disturbed. Don't let the tail end of something cut into your time.

4. Use the fifteen-minute rule for those times when you really don't feel like practicing. Make it the ten-minute rule if you're really squeamish. Resolve to start. You'll stay for only fifteen minutes. Then if you don't want to continue, you'll stop at fifteen minutes. See how you feel after fifteen. I bet you'll stay longer.

5. Have a plan B. If you're tackling a really hard practice, maybe with a lot of strength training, give yourself an alternative with lots of relaxation or inner work. And vice versa, if you're embroiled in a huge piece of inner work that seems to be going on and on, give yourself a straightforward basic practice with no errand into the maze.

There are going to be days when life gets the best of you. You can't get the practice in even though you tried! Here are some mini-practices that my clients and I use (more often than I wish) that give some of yoga's benefits and keep us practicing. Even though they're brief, when I do them I feel my practice continues and I haven't lost the thread. It's far easier to shrink and expand an existing practice than to start one up again.

THE 15-MINUTE QUICKIE PRACTICE

❊ Solar Energizer (*Agni Sara*)

❊ Sun Salutation (*Surya Namaskara*)

❊ Half Moon Pose (*Ardha Chandrasana*)

✳ Downward-Facing Boat Pose (*Navasana*)

✳ Posterior Stretch Pose (*Paschimottanasana*)

✳ Half Spinal Twist Pose (*Ardha Matsyendrasana*)

✳ Shoulder Stand Pose (*Sarvangasana*), Plow Pose (*Halasana*), Half Fish Pose (*Ardha Matsyasana*)

✳ Relaxation in Basic Relaxation Pose (*Shavasana*)

THE STUCK-IN-A-CHAIR OFFICE PRACTICE

✳ While seated, bend back and then forward like in the Sun Salutation (*Surya Namaskara*)

✳ Elbows Cross in Front

✳ Clasp—One Up, One Down

✳ Clasp—Behind Back

✳ Sitting Side Bend with Neck Work (*Parshvottanasana*)

✳ Sitting Twist Pose (*Bharadvajasana*) using chair arm or back

✳ Relax—Fold arms on desk and place forehead on backs of wrists

THE GO TO SLEEP PRACTICE

This practice works if you do all the steps in order:

Step 1. Do 5 to 10 minutes of Alternate Nostril Breathing (*Nadi Shodhanam*)

Step 2. Chant "Om" for 3 minutes (If it's hard to sit comfortably to do this, lie down.)

Step 3. Get in bed, lie on your back. Take seven breaths with 2-to-1 Ratioed Breathing (that is, exhale is twice as long as the inhale). Turn to your left side. Take seven more 2-to-1 ratioed breaths. Turn to your right side. Take seven more ratioed breaths. If you are still awake, repeat this again.

THE WALKING *PRANAYAMA* PRACTICE

You're at a conference with colleagues or staying in close quarters with in-laws who'll think you have a screw loose if you get down in front of the big screen TV for some pelvic centering poses! You can, however, go for a walk, and in the time you're out there (away from it all—yea!), do some yogic breathing as you stroll. Here's a gem of a practice from Sri Swami Sivananda. Take a thirty-minute walk and do this breathing practice during the beginning, middle, and end of the time you spend walking. Breathe in and count as you take each step: 1, 2, 3, 4. Breathe out and count: 1, 2, 3, 4. When this is comfortable, extend the length of your exhale to six counts, so that you breathe in for four and out for six. You may find you can extend the count to six counts as you inhale and nine counts as you exhale or even more. Just keep the same ratio of 1-to-1-½. Try to get this in twice a day. As you improve, see how much of the thirty minutes can be done with this ratioed *pranayama*. Once you've mastered thirty minutes, go for one hour.

THE SOLAR ENERGIZER (*AGNI SARA*)

Sri Swami Rama of the Himalayas was noted for suggesting "yoga first-aid" in the form of the Solar Energizer (*Agni Sara*) if you don't have time to do a longer Hatha Yoga practice. Begin with ten repetitions per session, making sure your stomach is empty. Gradually work up to twenty-five repetitions. Shoot for twice a day. This practice will help keep your digestive system toned and your internal organs healthy. Skip it when you're menstruating or pregnant or if you have high blood pressure. See the details on *Agni Sara* in chapter 3.

PRACTICE "BOTH/AND" TO RIDE OUT CHANGE

Many of us are first exposed to yoga through a class that offers a single repetitive routine of postures. This is like learning to cook using only one recipe. When you delve further into yoga, you become a chef who can cook anything. We may initially be attracted to yoga's fitness aspect. Yet in terms of what yoga has to offer, this is merely an introduction that cracks open the door, enabling us to peer into a world of unshakable faith, compassion, and liberation.

Your yoga practice will be most satisfying over the long haul if you work from both sides of the continuum. At times, make it exactingly rigorous; at other times, allow it to be intuitively open to possibility. Advertisers display images of women who appear perfect. Hatha Yoga practice has the potential to bring your body to a state of maximal health. But if we seek perfection at the cost of wholeness, we unconsciously unleash nature's powers of equilibrium in our psyche. Practicing in a way that is not driven by a merciless bully but is open to the opinion of every part of you will allow you to continuously reestablish dynamic equilibrium at every level of your being throughout your life.

There is a story of a master weaver of Persian rugs who wove carpets of the most fabulously intricate design. The oddity was that he purposefully made one small error in each work. When asked why one as capable as he would invite this imperfection, he replied, "The mistake is the place where the soul enters the work." Hold a space for the things in your body, behavior, relationships, and thinking that aren't working for you. Take them onto your lap and rock them. Give them voice so the façade of perfection can fade into an honest life enriched by the melodies of your soul.

Once the great *Jnana* yogi Sri Nisargadatta Maharaj was asked if he was ever perturbed by all the things that go wrong in life. He remarked that he was never perturbed by dissonance, but rather was astounded that human nature insists on believing everything is going to run smoothly and precisely as we expect. As one teacher put it, if you have a good diet, have slept well, and have no problems, your practice will be perfect every day. But alas, life is full of surprises, and we can't control everything that comes our way. Yoga practice helps us ride life's unforeseeable and inevitable changes. Creating a yogic lifestyle by mindfully choosing options that support health and self-understanding is the topic of the next and final chapter.

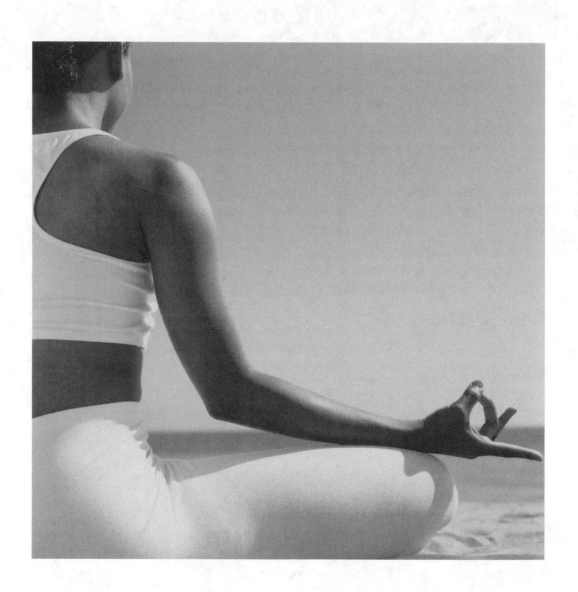

chapter 12

the other twenty-three hours: a yogic guide to the rest of your life

We must be the change we wish to see.
—Mohandas Gandhi

And I have asked to be
Where no storms come,
Where the green swell is in the havens dumb,
And out of the swing of the sea.

—From "A Nun Takes the Veil,"
Gerard Manley Hopkins

In "A Nun Takes the Veil," Gerard Manley Hopkins depicts monastic life's ability to minimize the distraction and interruption implicit in worldly affairs. A spiritual center such as a monastery or yoga ashram provides community, structure, and routine, which stabilizes the life rhythms of residents. It may also focus on regulating diet and exercise. This is why time spent at a yoga retreat center helps your practice get off on the right foot and supports your continuing commitment to it. Since most of us are not going to live our lives "out of the swing of the sea," we need to find ways to keep an even keel in order to make progress in the thick of it all. "Be like the lotus flower: its roots are in the mud, yet it blossoms above the water," booms Sri Swami Rama. "Live in the world but rise above it." A peaceful life lived in harmony with nature is the yogic ideal. This is accomplished through discrimination and conservation.

lifestyle diet

The word *diet* usually refers to controlling the intake of food. But what if we expand its meaning to include anything we take in and absorb? Our *lifestyle diet* consists of whatever we engage in throughout each day. Each activity and each interaction, from one with our boss, our spouse, or the gas station attendant, leaves an impression. Our body chemistry is constantly responding to our thoughts and feelings. Every single thought played upon our mental screen causes some bodily reaction. While there are unavoidable events in life, and at times the right action is to charge headlong into conflict, yoga advises us to carefully consider the effects of our worldly interactions. This is not only to promote amenable interchange, but to reduce the sheer amount of discord we wittingly, or habitually and unwittingly, invite into our experience.

Examine your lifestyle diet in terms of three overlapping areas. See how you are affected emotionally, mentally, and energetically by the different events and interchanges in your day. Because of their prevalence and importance in our lives, relationships are an important place to begin. Choose a current relationship and ask yourself, "What effect does this person tend to have on my energy and emotions?" Ask "What thoughts predominate when I spend time with her or him?" Our family friend Henrietta is energetically uplifting. Her energy is so bright and her emotions are so pleasant that even our very shy cat comes out to sit by her feet. On the other hand, my mother has a friend who focuses on morbid details.

Whenever this woman visits, she tells vivid stories of horrible accidents and life crises. When she leaves, I can almost see the dense emotional atmosphere left by her words in the air. Maybe you know someone—a friend, relative, or colleague—who draws you into her negative thought patterns. You meet for dinner. You start off happy enough, but her negative mind-set permeates every aspect of conversation. By the end of the evening, you leave grumbling about something you aren't even involved in, or are mad at your husband because she's mad at hers!

Satsang is a Sanskrit word that means "in the company of truth." Individuals who are on a program of self-improvement often find that they are most comfortable and progress more quickly when they keep the company of others with similar aims. This is one reason why individuals in groups such as AA succeed. Like-minded people support one another. Ancient yogis described thoughts as waves, called *vrittis*. If we desire a calm mind and a life of focused intention, we'll seek a personal environment and way of interacting that reduce mental and emotional turbulence. When we get carried off on turbulent mental waves and charged-up emotions, we waste loads of energy. This doesn't mean we need to dump all our friends because they're not perfect. However, yoga does advise us to become aware of how our relationships affect us and to discriminate based on this personal research. We may develop the capacity to tolerate, redirect, or offer support to those we encounter. There are also times when we must let go.

An area of "mental diet" that can subtly pull us into negativity is exposure to violent, upsetting, or overwhelming images from advertisers and the entertainment industry. If you live in Western culture, such images are embedded in your everyday life. As your yoga practice progresses, you may notice greater sensitivity to the effect of these images on your nervous system. You'll certainly become more conscious of their effect on your mind. As you continue with yoga, you may choose to eliminate voluntary exposure to extreme images that disturb your mind and induce a stressful response in your body. Of course, there is a point at which you become so firmly established in your indwelling Self that you're no longer vulnerable to these triflings. Perhaps this is true for you now.

silence (maunam)

If you wonder why lifestyle dieting is important to your health, spend some time in silence. In keeping silent we come to hear the noisiness of our own mind. The yoga practice of withholding speech (*maunam*) can be taken on for any length of time. A full day without speech works well as a unit of time in which to try this out. Not able to devote this much time? Try the practice for several hours. If you're the hub of many wheels, you may need to communicate now and then throughout your period of silence. Use a small chalkboard for this. If you find yourself continuously scribbling messages, reconsider either the chalkboard or the practice itself.

If a period of silence is completely out of the question just now, you can practice the essence of silence without completely eliminating speech by deciding to use words sparingly for a period of time. Tell significant others what you're up to beforehand.

These practices reveal the normal busy chatter of your mind. They help you see your thoughts for what they are: waves on the surface of the ocean of the mind. As you become quieter externally, you find a strong connection to the quiet place within you. Resorting to this quiet place, you can see the patterns of your personality and emotions as if you were sitting in a movie theater and watching a dramatic story unfold. From this vantage point, you can clearly determine which input and expenditures of energy are worth your while and which you would be better without. A period of silence has the benefit of refining your discrimination in terms of when, how, and with whom you're willing to engage.

the seven treasures of balanced health

Of equal importance to filtering what we take in is stabilizing our natural rhythms. There's an old saying: "Nature, to be commanded, must be obeyed." If you want to examine your health for factors that cause or contribute to imbalance, look at how close to nature you're living. Yoga offers a life-boosting strategy that creates and maintains health through guidance in several lifestyle areas. I call these areas the Seven Treasures of Balanced Health. Each one is a pillar in the palace of your vitality. I will go so far as to say that most cases of disease begin as a seed of imbalance in one of these areas. Use the Seven Treasures as a guide to examine your lifestyle. What do you do on a day-to-day basis to support your health, and what do you do to challenge it?

TREASURE 1. REGULARITY AND ROUTINE

We are creatures of habit. Do something for a few days running, and when you stop, you miss it. Since whatever we do repeatedly is going to stick anyway, we may as well consciously choose habits that support health and keep us in sync with nature's rhythms. If we respect nature's cycles, she will reward us with balanced health, considerable endurance, and a storehouse of vitality.

The Four Fountains

Yoga identifies four inherent fountains in all living beings. They are primitive drives that serve our health best when regulated by routine. Naturally, there will be times when you live off the clock. But even these times will be sustainable because of the time you have spent following a regular routine. A regular, natural rhythm is a major cornerstone of balanced health.

Sleep, the first drive, is recommended when there is no light in the sky. On a regular basis, get as close to waking with daylight and sleeping with darkness as you can. Cut out staying up all hours to be overstimulated by the entertainment industry's barrage of extreme imagery. At the very least, get up and go to bed at the same time each ordinary day.

Hunger is the next fountain. Eating at regular times in a pleasant atmosphere and in an unhurried way will aid digestion and allow you to pay attention. There is a saying that food turns to poison if eaten in haste, when you're exhausted, or under emotional duress. If possible, try to make your main meal at noon. This isn't just to avoid weight gain; it's to effectively utilize your digestive fire, which peaks at midday when the sun is highest.

The third fountain is *sex*. You may have heard the locker room stories about athletes swearing off sex during their competitive season. Too much sexual interaction depletes vitality, just as bearing many children does. While applying the word *routine* to sexuality seems boring, keeping sexual fulfillment at bay to allow for a crescendo of desire and a depth to satiation is one result of regulated abstinence.

Self-preservation is the fourth fountain. And while we're not concerned with being eaten by a tiger, we may come across one in the boardroom. When we're stressed and overworked, when our habit is to push ourselves all the time, we initiate a fight-flight reaction in our neuro-endocrine system. If we keep this pattern in place over time, we use up our reserves, making withdrawals without any deposits. With the upsurge of coffeehouses across the United States, we see this pattern as the modus operandi of our time. It's an insidious pattern of expenditure that will eventually take its toll. Keeping a doable routine to our days is a long-term pillar of health. Ask yourself how busy you are and how much of this is self-created. What can you let go? Do you need to change jobs, delegate, or have a talk with your superior about workload? Do you need to find a baby-sitter? Find recreational activities that balance your work actions. If you sit at a computer all day, don't go home and surf the Net. Get outside and move! Break up your day with counterbalancing yoga movement breaks. Make them part of your routine so you'll miss them if you don't do them. They'll become the mortar in your palace of good health.

TREASURE 2. ADEQUATE REST

I'm not going to tell you to get eight hours—but winding down before bed, doing a few poses and some breathing practices, can support your "digestion" of the day, sending you off to dreamland relaxed and ready to let go. Alternate nostril breathing will help balance the nervous system, as will a few minutes of optimal diaphragmatic breathing while relaxing on your back. You might decide that meditation practice would be useful here as well. Try setting aside a half hour to an hour to slow down and get ready for sleep. You'll sleep well and wake refreshed. (Also see the Go to Sleep practice in chapter 11.)

Take breaks throughout the day to press your "reset" button. Be aware of your stress level, and seek recuperative activities to reduce it. My friend Steve simply walks to the water fountain. He stays hydrated, he moves a bit, stretches some, looks out the window to relax his eyes, and he's back in the saddle. It doesn't take much. Before I began my own business, my boss and I used to close the door to her office for a few minutes before lunch to take a diaphragmatic breathing break. Our office resembled Grand Central most of the day, with people bustling in and out. We'd turn off the lights and rest on the floor in the Corpse Pose to breathe. We wouldn't talk or remind one another of things to get done; we'd simply take a true break, rest on our backs, and attend to even breathing for about ten minutes.

You may not be able to lie on your boss's floor, but see if you can incorporate some yoga rest breaks into your day. Lisé uses her computer's downloading time to remember to slow her breathing. You'll be surprised by how much clarity of focus and restored energy just a few moments provide.

TREASURE 3. FRESH AND NATURAL FOOD

In food we are looking for *prana*, vital energy. Forget for a moment about protein, carbohydrates, and fat, and think that to maintain life you want to take in life. You want to eat food that has as much life in it when you eat it as possible! Fresh fruits and vegetables in balance with grains and legumes should make up the main portion of your diet. Whether you eat meat or not, strive to make your diet plant-based and the freshest you can find. Preparing and eating leafy greens fresh from the market should become part of your daily life. Have raw food every day, such as salad, fruit, a smoothie, fresh vegetable juice. When you cook vegetables, do it with the minimal amount of heat and until they're just done, so they're as close to their natural state as possible. This not only retains higher vitamin and mineral content; it retains *prana*. If you can't get fresh, choose frozen over canned. Avoid highly processed foods and foods with lots of additives.

Look for variety in your menu. Use a host of ingredients in your salads. Try new vegetables and combinations of legumes and grains. Variety in food choices gives you the greatest chance of getting all the vitamins, minerals, balanced proteins, carbohydrates, and fats you need without supplements.

Take vitamin and mineral supplements when you recognize you haven't been supplying your body with balanced nutrition and during particularly hectic times. If you take supplements daily, you might want to take some time off from them to explore getting all the nutrition you need just from food. This gives your body a chance to rid itself of things you've been taking that it doesn't need.

Use your body to know what to eat. Smell the food and pay attention to your gut response. If you get a strong physical response to put the food directly into your mouth, then it's likely to be something you need. If you want to eat something because you have it every day or because you just saw it on TV, give it the sniff test. When you smell this food, does your gut say, "Yes, eat it now"? Is there a so-so feeling or even a slight repulsion? Can you forgo this food choice and check in with your hunger? Notice your inner dialogue and what comes into your awareness when you choose this option.

After eating, study the effect of the food on your state of being. Did the meal leave you feeling focused and energized, dull, or hyper? Make note of which foods leave you energized, clear-headed, and able to focus.

TREASURE 4. CLEANSING

Internal cleansing is an often overlooked aspect of health in the West. A daily fast is universally recommended, taking place from the end of your light evening meal at around seven until you have breakfast the next morning. Cutting out evening (or any) snacking will give your digestive system a chance to get through its "In Box" before you add more work. It may even get rid of some excess. Skip an occasional meal. Hunger is a sign of increased *agni* or digestive fire and an excellent way of metabolizing the excess that impedes health.

A moderately strenuous Hatha Yoga practice will cause you to perspire, as will a brisk walk. Activities that use less than 50 percent of your total available energy will not deplete reserves, yet get the juices flowing. This helps to move waste and toxins out of your body. Performing *Agni Sara* and other heating practices gives similar benefits and further stimulates your digestive and eliminatory systems.

Vigorously brushing your skin with a dry skin brush for several minutes each day will tone this organ of elimination. Wearing synthetic clothing that doesn't breathe holds the toxins released through your pores against your skin, where they're reabsorbed. The skin drinks what you put on it, so wear natural fiber clothes for evaporation and use natural oils and lotions. A rule of thumb is, "Don't put anything on your skin you wouldn't want to eat," because it will end up inside your body.

Water was used as an ancient cure, with methods handed down for thousands of years. Drink four to ten large glasses of water throughout the day, depending on the weather and whether the food you eat is juicy or salty. Make hot or cold water packs by soaking folded pads of flannel or other natural fabrics in water and apply them to your skin for a localized tissue cleansing. The water will be taken into the body as the toxins under the skin are drawn out.

Yoga has other purification methods (*kriyas*) to help eliminate mucus, toxins, and other impurities from the body. The nasal wash (*jala neti*) and the upper wash (*gajakarani*) don't require personal instruction.

In the nasal wash, water is used to clean the nostrils of germ-catching mucus and dirt. This can prevent colds and alleviate allergy symptoms. You can do this practice in the morning and evening and more frequently when you are congested. When your nasal passageways are blocked or your mucus membranes are covered with impurities, your nose can't perform its functions effectively. In the nasal wash, a small pot is used to pour water from one nostril to the other and from each nostril to the mouth. The pot is filled with warm salt water and poured over a sink or basin.

In the stomach wash, warm saltwater is used to cleanse the digestive tract from the stomach to the mouth. The stomach wash (*gajakarani*) is done by drinking a large quantity of warm salty water until the stomach is full and then vomiting it out by tickling the back of the throat. Most of the difficulty with this practice is that we associate it with the feeling of being nauseous. When we're sick, vomiting is an involuntary natural process our body uses as a last resort. When done voluntarily with only saltwater, the noxious aspects are eliminated and the practice becomes agreeable.

The bowels can be cleansed through fasting, water drinking, herbal and dietary supplements in conjunction with or without Hatha Yoga postures, and enemas. Bowel cleansing is an important aspect of yogic cleansing, for which

nasal wash (*jala neti*)

1. Use ½ cup or more of warm water with about ⅛ teaspoon of salt added. It should taste as salty as a teardrop.

2. Put this solution in a *neti* pot, which looks like a miniature teapot with a long spout, or use any sort of small container that has a spout.

3. Stand over a sink and slightly tilt your head to one side. Place the spout in your higher nostril and pour the water into it. If your head is in the right position, the water will drain out the lower nostril. Repeat on the other side.

4. With this practice you can also clean the passageway from each nostril to the mouth. As you tilt your head to the side and begin to pour the water, sniff the water into your nose. Then allow it to come out of your mouth. Do this on the other side.

stomach wash (*gajakarani*)

1. Mix salt into four to six quarts of warm water. It should taste like the ocean.

2. On an empty stomach, drink the water as quickly as possible, keeping your torso upright.

3. When you can't take in another drop, lean forward over the toilet (or do this outside), and gently tickle the back of your throat. Repeat this until all the water has been expelled.

4. Refrain from eating any more than juice or fruit for a few hours afterward.

I suggest you seek experienced guidance. There are people who specialize in internal cleansing. A good place to begin looking for someone in your area is to ask your yoga teacher, chiropractor, or naturopathic physician. Also, centers such as the Himalayan Institute's Center for Health and Healing offer on-site programs with medical doctors and well-trained staff.

TREASURE 5. APPROPRIATE MOVEMENT AND EXERCISE

In addition to implementing yoga practice into your life, include some form of aerobic exercise. Walking, jogging, or cycling can be done outside in fresh air and sunlight and require a minimal amount of equipment. Some Hatha Yoga practices can be done for cardiovascular effect. However, unless you're in peak condition using optimal form, you may find the wear on your joints counterproductive.

Dancing can be a great aerobic workout. Music can be inspiring, freeing, empowering, and heart opening. Dance alone with the curtains drawn, outside among nature, with friends, your lover, your kids, or go out! Take a dance class or try a hybrid yoga dance class like Yogaerobics or DansKinetics. Throughout history, dance was used to mark major events in life and in the life of communities. You may decide to create movement rituals to mark changes you go through as a woman.

Experiment with movement practices that agree with you. Instead of just getting through it, tune in and experience the movement. If you get a little bored, focus on your technique just like in yoga practice. Feel your life force, listen to the rhythm of your breathing, inwardly sense your alignment. Keep your goals in mind, but respect your body's limitations and capacity to avoid creating mental resistance and physical injury. Experiment with movement practices that agree with you; then set aside time to enjoy them!

TREASURE 6. COUNTERACTING LIFESTYLE STRESS

Because life is a dynamic process, imbalances occur as par for the course. Yoga practice cultivates attentiveness to our sense of well-being so that when we first notice we're swinging too far off the normal curve, we can counterbalance to regain mental, emotional, energetic, or physical equilibrium. Yoga teaches us to seek recuperative situations so we don't become completely unbalanced and descend into illness.

Sometimes we can't immediately extricate ourselves from a harmful circumstance. For example, you find your work environment toxic, but need a job. So as you search for a new one while still holding down the old one, you balance that stress with activities that allow you to detoxify your body and mind. You don't hit the bar or the Dairy Queen, but instead run, kickbox, dance, or do vigorous Hatha Yoga so the body can flush out the negative feelings and chemical toxins. Otherwise, to compensate for the job stress, there's a danger you might adopt an addictive habit that will accelerate a spiral into illness, or you might become overwhelmed by negative influences that disturb your equilibrium in some other way.

Another thing that helps to balance life stress is to schedule time for your practice. One of Stephen Covey's best strategies for effective living is a category he calls "sharpening the saw." Instead of running around putting out fires, commit to making time for balancing self-care. Use the time for exercise, rest, play, relationship work, or whatever will provide balance. Sometimes the hardest part is seeing that you need to do it!

TREASURE 7. HARMONY OF SOUL

From yoga's point of view, mental and emotional digestion rate right up there with physical digestion. Keeping things flowing is critical for good health. If something is eating you, take care of it right away. Don't bury it, seize up, or close down. Don't let the fear of facing it keep you from being present or drive you away from taking necessary action. To me, the Sanskrit word *spanda* indicates the point at which an intention comes into form. When an intention comes into form, it is important to acknowledge it and not repress it. Becoming aware of the spontaneous assertions arriving in your psyche and body from beyond awareness is a meditative process. You may choose to enter this process in different ways; the important point is that you *do* enter the process.

As the *Bhagavad Gita* suggests, "Day after day, let the yogi practice the harmony of soul: in a secret place, in deep solitude, master of his mind, hoping for nothing, desiring nothing." In the case of sitting meditation, you witness the flow of *spanda*, events arising and dissipating while remaining centered in peace. Or you may choose to examine the assertions coming from within through your Hatha Yoga or movement practice. Part Three of this book, "Soul Yoga: Look Within," is devoted to options you can use to explore *spanda*. Pay attention to signals your soul sends through your body, imagination, dreams, preferences, and relationships. Pay attention to synchronicities and the odd events in your world. Then use your own yoga practice to process what you perceive. Let inspiration move you into appropriate action. If the course of action is not yet clear to you, stay present to the flow of your process. However you choose to work with yourself, you must give yourself time to arrive at a place of quiet focus.

Although the irrational isn't ruled by reason, it's not invalid! Don't allow the prevalent rationalistic worldview to rob you of a richly textured and intriguing life. Women are gifted with significant intuitive power. Use yours. By owning our gifts, we create a field-like network of compassionate individuals who peacefully acquire the power to redirect the severe imbalance in our world. The strength of this collective does not come from a top-heavy position of authority or control, but from a grounded sense of connection with all life.

Service, or *seva*, as it is called in Sanskrit, is one of humanity's most powerful self-help practices. It restores and fortifies inner harmony when done without compulsion or guilt. Service loosens our attachment to being in control and having things our way. Giving generously to those less fortunate or to a worthy cause helps us disentangle from desires and from our conceptual grip on reality. As we let go of the fabrication of who we are, we are free to realize the universal Spirit within.

above all

At this pause in our relationship, I hope you will make whatever is useful to you in these pages your own. Don't worry if you goof up. Everybody does! Just begin again. Know that people like you and me are beginning over and over again, too. Study your response to the work, trust yourself, adapt the practices. As the starship captain played by Tim Allen in the hilarious movie *Galaxy Quest* regales, "Never give up, never surrender!" Every single positive action you take will result in something positive in your life, which in turn gives your practice momentum. Finally, I wish for you Sri Nisargadatta Maharaj's experience of yoga's goal:

> Above all, infinite affection, love, dark and quiet, radiating in all directions, embracing all, making all interesting and beautiful, significant and auspicious.

appendix A: yoga books

While these resources have a sensibility similar to *Every Woman's Yoga*, they will take you further in the direction of interest their titles suggest.

Anderson, Sandra & Rolf Sovik. *Yoga: Mastering the Basics.* Himalayan Institute, Honesdale, PA, 2000.

Ballentine, Rudolph, M.D. *Diet and Nutrition: A Holistic Approach.* Himalayan Institute, Honesdale, PA, 1978.

Ballentine, Rudolph, M.D. *Radical Healing.* Harmony Books, New York, 1999.

Ballentine, Rudolph, M.D. *The Theory and Practice of Meditation.* Himalayan Institute, Honesdale, PA, 1986.

Bohm, David. *Wholeness and the Implicate Order.* Ark, Routledge and Kegan Paul Ltd., London, 1983.

Chödrön, Pema. *When Things Fall Apart: Heart Advice for Difficult Times.* Shambhala, Boston, 1997.

Chopra, Deepak, M.D. *Perfect Weight: The Complete Mind/Body Program for Achieving and Maintaining Your Ideal Weight.* Harmony Books, New York, 1994.

Chopra, Deepak. *Quantum Healing: Exploring the Frontiers of Mind/Body Medicine.* Bantam Books, New York, 1989.

Cohen, Bonnie Bainbridge. *Sensing, Feeling, and Action: The Experiential Anatomy of Body-Mind Centering.* Contact Editions, Northampton, MA, 1993.

Chopra, Deepak. *Perfect Health: The Complete Mind/Body Guide.* Harmony Books, New York, 1991.

Coulter, H. David. *Anatomy of Hatha Yoga: A Manual for Students, Teachers and Practitioners.* Body and Breath, Honesdale, PA 2001.

Dworkis, Sam. *Recovery Yoga: A Practical Guide for Chronically Ill, Injured, and Post-Operative People*. Three Rivers Press, New York, 1997.

Estes, Clarissa Pinkola. *Women Who Run with the Wolves: Myths and Stories of the Wild Woman Archetype*. Ballantine Books, New York, 1992.

Farhi, Donna. *The Breathing Book: Good Health and Vitality Through Essential Breath Work*. Henry Holt and Company, New York, 1996.

Farhi, Donna. *Yoga Mind Body and Spirit: A Return to Wholeness*. Henry Holt and Company, New York, 2000.

Huber, Cheri. *There is Nothing Wrong with You*. Keep It Simple Books, Mountain View, CA 1993.

Jensen, Bernard, D.C. *Doctor-Patient Handbook: Dealing with the Reversal Process and the Healing Crisis Through Eliminating Diets and Detoxification*. Bernard Jensen International, Escondido, CA, 196.

Jensen, Bernard, D.C. *Tissue Cleansing Through Bowel Management*. Bernard Jensen Enterprises, Escondido, CA 1981.

Knaster, Mirka. *Discovering the Body's Wisdom*. Bantam, New York, 1996.

Lad, Vasant. *Ayurveda: The Science of Self Healing*. Lotus Press, Santa Fe, NM, 1984.

Lasater, Judith. *Relax and Renew: Restful Yoga for Stressful Times*. Rodmell Press, Berkeley, CA, 1995.

Mindell, Arnold. *Dreambody: The Body's Role in Revealing the Self*. Sigo Press, Boston, 1982.

Mindell, Arnold. *Working on Yourself Alone: Inner Dreambody Work*. Arkane, London, 1990.

Mindell, Arnold. *Working with the Dreaming Body*. Routledge and Kegan Paul, London, 1987.

Moore, Thomas. *Care of the Soul*. Harper Perennial, New York, 1994.

Moore, Thomas. *Original Self: Living with Paradox and Originality*. Perennial, New York, 2001.

Murray, Michael, N.D. and Joseph Pizzorno, N.D. *Encyclopedia of Natural Medicine*. Prima, Rocklin, CA 1991.

Noble, Elizabeth. *Essential Exercises for the Childbearing Year: A Guide to Health and Comfort Before and After Your Baby is Born*. New Life Images, Harwich, MA, 1995.

Northrup, Christiane, M.D. *The Wisdom of Menopause: Creating Physical and Emotional Health and Healing During the Change*. Bantam, New York, 2001.

Northrup, Christiane, M.D. *Women's Bodies, Women's Wisdom: Creating Physical and Emotional Health and Healing*. Bantam, New York, 1998.

Nuernberger, Phil. *Freedom from Stress*. Himalayan Institute, Honesdale, PA 1981.

Ojeda, Linda. *Menopause without Medicine*. Hunter House, Inc. Alameda, CA, 1995.

Olsen, Andrea, with Caryn McHose. *Bodystories: A Guide to Experiential Anatomy*. Station Hill Press, Barrytown, NY, 1991.

Pelletier, Kenneth R. *Mind as Healer, Mind as Slayer*. Delta, New York, 1977.

Pitchford, Paul. *Healing with Whole Foods: Oriental Traditions and Modern Nutrition*. North Atlantic Books, Berkeley, CA, 1993.

Pizzorno, Joseph, N.D. *Total Wellness: Improve Your Health by Understanding the Body's Healing Systems*. Prima Publishing, Rocklin, CA, 1996.

Raichur, Pratima. *Absolute Beauty: Radiant Skin and Inner Harmony Through the Ancient Secrets of Ayurveda*. Harper Perennial, New York, 1997.

Rama, Swami. *Meditation and Its Practice*. Himalayan Institute, Honesdale, PA 1992.

Rama, Swami and Swami Ajaya. *Creative Use of Emotions*. Himalayan Institute, Honesdale, PA 1979.

Rama, Swami, Rudolph Ballentine, and Swami Ajaya. *Yoga and Psychotherapy: The Evolution of Consciousness*. Himalayan Institute, Honesdale, PA 1976.

Rama, Swami, Rudolph Ballentine, Alan Hymes. *Science of Breath: A Practical Guide*. Himalayan Institute, Honesdale, PA 1988.

Ramaswami, Srivatsa. *Yoga for the Three Stages of Life: Developing Your Practice as an Art Form, a Physical Therapy, and a Guiding Philosophy*. Inner Traditions, Rochester, VT, 2000.

Schiffmann, Erich. *Yoga: The Spirit and Practice of Moving into Stillness*. Pocket Books, New York, 1996.

Schulz, Mona Lisa, M.D., Ph.D. *Awakening Intuition: Using Your Mind-Body Network for Insight and Healing*. Three Rivers Press, New York, 1998.

Svoboda, Robert. *Ayurveda for Women: A Guide to Vitality and Health*. David and Charles, Devon, England, 1999.

Svoboda, Robert. *Ayurveda: Life, Health and Longevity*. Penguin, London, 1992.

Svoboda, Robert. *Prakruti: Your Ayurvedic Constitution*. Geocom, Albuquerque, MN, 1988.

Tigunait, Pandit Rajmani. *Inner Quest: The Path of Spiritual Unfoldment*. Yoga International Books, Honesdale, PA, 1995.

Tigunait, Pandit Rajmani. *The Power of Mantra and the Mystery of Initiation*. Himalayan Institute, Honesdale, PA, 1996.

Tiwari, Maya. *Ayurveda: Secrets of Healing*. Lotus Press, Twin Lakes, WI, 1995.

Tiwari, Bri. Maya. *The Path of Practice: A Woman's Book of Healing with Food, Breath, and Sound*. Ballantine, New York, 2000.

Walton, Todd. *Open Body: Creating Your Own Yoga*. Avon, New York, 1998.

Weil, Andrew, M.D. *Eating Well for Optimum Health*. Alfred A. Knopf, New York, 2000.

Weil, Andrew, M.D. *Eight Weeks to Optimal Health: A Proven Program for Taking Advantage of Your Body's Natural Healing Power*. Ballantine, New York, 1997.

Weil, Andrew, M.D. *Spontaneous Healing: How to Discover and Enhance Your Body's Natural Ability to Maintain and Heal Itself*. Ballantine, New York, 1995.

appendix B: yoga videos

After I had my second child, we moved into a tiny cabin in a mountainous region and got 14 inches of snow that stayed on the ground until the end of April! I had little to spare for a creative practice, so I resorted to following yoga videos until I could get more sleep and get out of the house! There are tons of videos on the market but who can see them all? My colleagues, students, clients, and I have used every one of these. They'll give you a good "class" by an expert teacher.

Crawford, Colette. *Postnatal Yoga with Colette Crawford*. Holistic Life Productions, 2000. (206) 525-9035.

Crawford, Colette. *Yoga for Pregnancy, Labor, and Birth*. Seattle Holistic Center, 2002. (206) 525-9035.

Farmer, Angela. *The Feminine Unfolding*. Transmit Media, Hohokus, NJ, 1999. (800) 343-5540. This is not a yoga class, but is definitely worth seeing.

Folan, Lilias. *Lilias! New Yoga—Total Body Workout for Beginners*. Cardio Challenge and Serenity Now, Natural Journeys, 2000. (800) 737-1825.

Folan, Lilias. *Lilias! New Yoga—Target Toning for Beginners*. Arms and Abs and Legs and Buns. Goldhil Home Media, 2000. (800) 250-8760 or (800) 737-1825.

Folan, Lilias. *Lilias! Discover Seniors Yoga: AM and PM*. Goldhil Home Media, 2002. (800) 250-8760 or (800) 737-1825.

Kripalu Yoga for Beginners Led by Stephen Cope. Kripalu Center, Lenox, MA 1994. (888) 399-1332.

Kripalu Yoga Dynamic Lead by Stephen Cope. Kripalu Yoga Fellowship, Lenox, MA 1998. (888) 399-1332.

Kripalu Yoga Gentle with Carolyn Lundeen. Kripalu Yoga Fellowship, Lenox, MA 1998. (888) 399-1332.

Yoga Breathing and Relaxation with Richard Freeman: An Introduction to the Internal Practice of Ashtanga Yoga. Delphi Productions, Ltd., 1997. (303) 443-2100.

Yoga at Home with Yogi Hari: For Radiant Health and Well Being. Sampoorna Hatha Yoga—Beginners Level 1, Beginners Level 2, Intermediate Level 1, Intermediate Level 2, and Advanced Level 1. Nada Productions, Ft. Lauderdale, FL, 1990. (800) 964-2553.

Yoga: Mastering the Basics: Deepen and Strengthen. Himalayan Institute, Honesdale, PA, 2000. (800) 822-4547.

Yoga: Mastering the Basics: Flexibility, Strength, and Balance. Himalayan Institute, Honesdale, PA, 2000. (800) 822-4547.

appendix C: places for yoga

Some of these centers are yoga ashrams, which are somewhat like monasteries. Whether you go for a weekend, a month, or longer, you join the routine of the place—getting up early, doing group practice, meditating, and possibly helping out in the kitchen. Other places listed here are retreat settings that offer a wide variety of programs including yoga.

The Expanding Light Retreat
14681 Tyler Foote Road, Nevada City, CA 95959
(800) 346-5350
www.expandinglight.org

Feathered Pipe Foundation
P.O. Box 1682, Helena, MT 59624
(406) 442-8196
www.featheredpipe.com

Himalayan Institute of Yoga Science and Philosophy
RR1, Box 400, Honesdale, PA 18431
(800) 822-4547
www.himalayaninstitute.org

Kripalu Center for Yoga and Health
P.O. Box 793, West Street, Rte. 183, Lenox, MA 01240
(800) 741-7353
www.kripalu.org

Mount Madonna Center
445 Summit Road, Watsonville, CA 95076
(408) 847-0406
www.mountmadonna.org

Omega Institute for Holistic Studies
150 Lake Drive, Rhinebeck, NY 12572-3212
(800) 944-1001
www.eomega.org

Satchidananda Ashram—Yogaville
Rte. 1, Box 1720, Buckingham, VA 23921
(800) 858-9642
www.yogaville.org

Sivananda Ashram Yoga Farm
14651 Ballantree Lane, Grass Valley, CA 95949
(800) 469-9642
www.sivananda.org

Sivananda Yoga Ranch Colony
P.O. Box 195. Budd Road, Woodbury, NY 12788
(845) 436-6492
www.sivananda.org

Yasodhara Ashram: Yoga Retreat and Study Centre
P.O. Box 9, Kootenay Bay, British Columbia, Canada V0B 1X0.
(800) 661-8711
www.yasodhara.org

appendix D: yoga stuff

Last Saturday, I walked into my neighborhood health food store and was greeted by a huge basket of brand new rolled yoga mats right next to the bread section—some weird baguettes? I thought. Your old sweatpants and T shirt, a bathrobe belt for a strap, and a really big book for a block are all you truly need. On the other hand, a few well chosen items up the aesthetic quotient and may help keep you motivated to practice. Yoga props, clothes, and paraphernalia are much more widely available than ever before. Many yoga centers and fitness studios have yoga supplies for sale, so check locally if you don't want to mail order. I've even seen "yoga stuff" in Wal-Mart and Old Navy. As in other places in this book, I am giving you varied options. Here are a few companies who have great customer service.

Age in Reverse
P.O. Box 1667, Newport Beach, CA 92663.
(888) AGE-EASY (243-3279) www.ageeasy.com

> *This is about inversion, so if doing the inverted poses is not possible, but it is safe for you to invert, these products are wonderful! Check out the Body Slant and the Body Lift.*

Bheka Yoga Supplies Company
258 A Street, #6, Ashland, OR 97520
(800) 366-4541 www.bheka.com.

> *A well-chosen selection. Check out the loose fitting Temple Pants.*

Gaiam, Inc.
360 Interlocken Blvd., Broomfield, CO 80021
(877) 989-6321 www.gaiam.com.

> *They have more than yoga supplies, calling themselves a lifestyle company.*

Maharishi Ayurveda Products International
1068 Elkton Drive, Colorado Springs, CO 80907
(800) 345-8332   www.mapi.com.

They carry a host of Ayurvedic products and help you select what is right for you.

Marie Wright Yoga Wear
1735 Olive Street, Santa Barbara, CA 93101.
(800) 217-0006   www.mariewright.net

For unitards and form fitting, yet comfortable clothing. Soft fabrics, great fit and colors.

Nature's Formulary,
14 Interstate Ave., Albany, NY 12205
(800) 923-9338, ext. 10   www.naturesformalary.com

They have Ayurvedic herbs like Triphala and Guggul.

Wellspring Homeopathic Pharmacy
(570) 253-5650

They'll mail order homeopathic remedies, herbs, and nutritional supplies and are extremely knowledgeable.

Yoga Pro
Box 7612, Ann Arbor, MI 48107
(800) 488-8414   www.yogapro.com

Check out the toe stretcher. A selection obviously based on serious practice.

*Yoga Zone
3342 Melrose Avenue, NW, Roanoke, VA 24017
800-264-9642   www.yogazone.com

Hot clothes, cool props.

appendix E:
sun salutation (Surya Namaskara)

1. Stand tall with hands at sides or at heart to prepare in Mountain Pose (*Tadasana*).

2. Raise arms overhead in Standing Staff Pose (*Samasthiti Dandasana*).

3. Arch backward into Backward-Bending Pose (*Urdhvasana*).

4. Return to Standing Staff Pose.

5. Fold over at hips into Standing Forward Fold Pose (*Uttanasara*).

6. Step one leg back into the lunging Monkey Pose (*Banarasara*) and arch upward.

7. Place palms on floor and touch toes, knees, chest, and nose to floor in Eight-Point Pose (*Ashtanamaskar*).

8. Arch upper body up and back into Upward-Facing Dog Pose (*Urdhva Mukha Shvanasara*).

9. Lift pelvis up and back into Downward-Facing Dog Pose (*Adho Mukha Shvanasara*).

10. Return to Monkey Pose (*Banarasara*).

11. Step feet together to return to Standing Forward Fold Pose (*Uttanasara*).

12. Return to standing with arms raised overhead in Standing Staff Pose (*Samasthiti Dardasara*).

13. Finish by bringing hands down or to the heart, or repeat by going directly into Backward-Bending Pose (*Urdhvasara*).

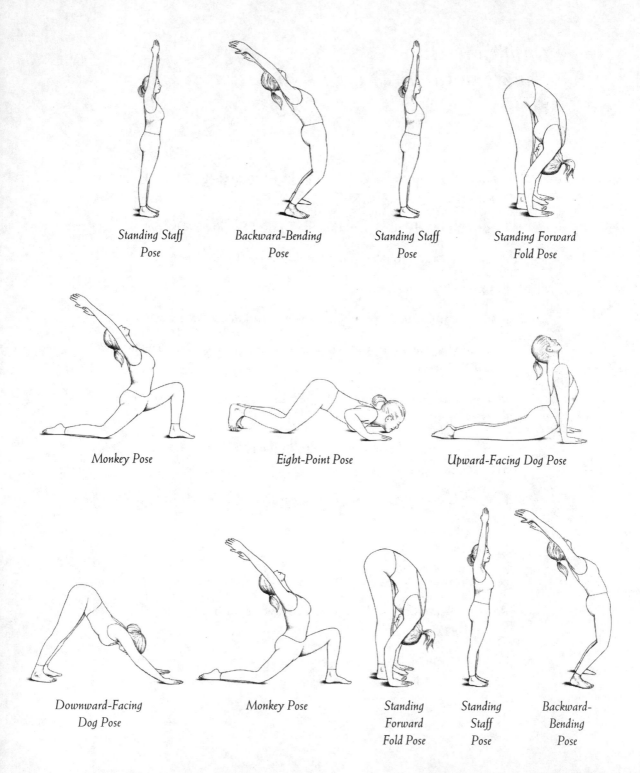

Standing Staff
Pose

Backward-Bending
Pose

Standing Staff
Pose

Standing Forward
Fold Pose

Monkey Pose

Eight-Point Pose

Upward-Facing Dog Pose

Downward-Facing
Dog Pose

Monkey Pose

Standing
Forward
Fold Pose

Standing
Staff
Pose

Backward-
Bending
Pose

pose index

index

about the author

Jaime Stover Schmitt, Ed. D., C.M.A., is the founder and president of Spanda: The Yoga of Movement—a private yoga movement therapy practice where she works with everyone from newborns to octogenarians—located in the New York metropolitan area. She began studying yoga at age 6 and has been teaching for almost 30 years.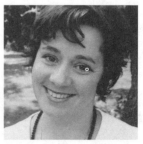

She received her doctoral degree in dance/movement studies from Temple University, in Philadelphia. Over the years she has gained vast and diverse training and experience in the arenas of movement/bodywork and yoga. At one point she studied in India under a master. Besides *Every Woman's Yoga*, Schmitt's most recent publication is *Yoga for Pregnancy* (Himalayan Institute Reprint Series, Himalayan Institute Press, 2001). She is also a contributor to *Yoga International Magazine*. Visit her Web site at www.spandayoga.com.